ADVANCE PRAISE FOR

GLUTEN-FREE
FAMILY FAVORITES

"Kelli and Peter Bronski offer us a wealth of recipes, designed with gluten-free families in mind. I love that this food is easy to make but still full of flavors. I want to make the Cashew Cream Scones, Breaded Zucchini Chips, and the Coconut Shrimp with Mango Dipping Sauce now! With three small children, the Bronskis know how to feed kids who need to live without gluten and get them involved in the cooking too."

—SHAUNA JAMES AHERN,
author of *Gluten-Free Girl Every Day* and *Gluten-Free Girl and the Chef:*
A Love Story with 100 Tempting Recipes

"The Bronskis excel at developing kid-friendly, gluten-free recipes, and the 75 dishes in Gluten-Free Family Favorites won't disappoint. But more than just a collection of delicious and nourishing recipes, Gluten-Free Family Favorites goes beyond, encouraging families to cook together as a means of bonding and forming healthy lifelong relationships with food. In a time when so many people are losing touch with their kitchens, I welcome Kelli and Peter's advice on empowering our children to take control of their health through cooking."

—LAURA B. RUSSELL,
author of *Brassicas* and *The Gluten-Free Asian Kitchen*

"For gluten-free households with children, it can be daunting to figure out what delicious dishes to safely serve everyone. The Bronskis have solved the problem with *Gluten-Free Family Favorites*. The gorgeous photos of every recipe invite you in and tempt you to preheat the oven immediately. And the recipes, such as French Toast Sticks, Sweet Potater Tots, Pupusa Pockets, Breaded Zucchini Chips, Soft Pretzels, and Apple Cider Donuts are not just tasty, but also offer allergen-free substitutions and a whole section on what kids can do to help. From the crash course in Gluten 101, to tips on supermarket savviness, to all the beautiful, fun-to-eat recipes, *Gluten-Free Family Favorites* is sure to become your most loved go-to cookbook."

—KYRA BUSSANICH,
author of *Sweet Cravings: 50 Seductive Desserts for the Gluten-Free Lifestyle*
and three-time Food Network *Cupcake Wars* champion

THE EXPERIMENT

BECAUSE EVERY BOOK IS A TEST OF NEW IDEAS

"I wish Peter and Kelli would adopt me into their family! Their focus on using familiar, accessible ingredients and clever recipe twists always yields flavorful food the whole family will enjoy."

—SILVANA NARDONE,
author of *Silvana's Gluten-Free and Dairy-Free Kitchen: Timeless Favorites Transformed* and *Cooking for Isaiah: Gluten-Free & Dairy-Free Recipes for Easy, Delicious Meals*

"*Gluten-Free Family Favorites* is a gift to those looking for recipes to feed the whole family, whether gluten-free or not. There's no weird food here, just good food that happens to be gluten-free. In addition to the scrumptious lineup of 75 recipes, several additional features set this book a step above the rest. Of particular note, the "Kids can . . ." sidebars are tremendously helpful. If you are just getting used to cooking gluten-free, or to cooking, period, you can certainly use the extra hands in the kitchen, and when kids help cook, they're guaranteed to eat it. Also significant are the alternatives at the foot of every recipe to help adapt these recipes to other dietary restrictions, such as dairy-free, nut-free, or vegan. While the recipes are notably kid-centric, they will appeal both to the kids and to the kid in all of us. These delicious home-style recipes are sure to keep your family happy, healthy, and busy in the kitchen for years to come."

—CYBELE PASCAL,
author of *Allergy-Free and Easy Cooking* and *The Allergen-Free Baker's Handbook* and founder of Cybele's Free-to-Eat

"If you have gluten-free kids, then you need this cookbook! Peter and Kelli teach the essentials of the gluten-free kitchen, plus share ways to get your little helpers involved. It is an invaluable resource for families living a gluten-free lifestyle, who not only want food that's nutritious and safe to eat, but also delicious meals that are truly enjoyable for everyone at the table (gluten-free or not). I know this is a cookbook that my family will use for years to come!"

—ALISON NEEDHAM,
founder of *A Girl Defloured*

KELLI AND PETER BRONSKI

GLUTEN-FREE
FAMILY FAVORITES

The 75 Go-To Recipes You Need to Feed Kids
and Adults All Day, Every Day

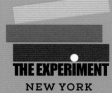

THE EXPERIMENT

NEW YORK

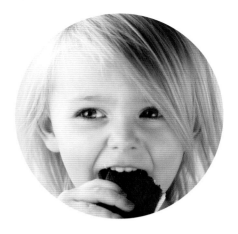

The Experiment, LLC
220 East 23rd Street, Suite 301
New York, NY 10010-4674
www.theexperimentpublishing.com

The Experiment's books are available at special discounts when purchased in bulk for premiums and sales promotions as well as for fund-raising or educational use. For details, contact us at info@theexperimentpublishing.com.

Gluten-Free Family Favorites includes a variety of gluten-free recipes as well as modifications including but not limited to refined-sugar-free, peanut-free, tree-nut-free, dairy-free, egg-free, and vegan alternatives. While care was taken to provide correct and helpful information, the suggestions in this book are not intended as dietary advice or as a substitute for consulting a dietician or medical professional. We strongly recommend that you check with your doctor before making changes to your diet. The authors and publisher disclaim all liability in connection with the use of this book.

Library of Congress Cataloging-in-Publication Data

Bronski, Kelli.
  Gluten-free family favorites : the 75 go-to recipes you need to feed kids and adults all day, every day / by Kelli and Peter Bronski.
     pages cm
  Includes bibliographical references and index.
  ISBN 978-1-61519-100-0 (pbk.) -- ISBN 978-1-61519-101-7 (ebook) 1. Gluten-free diet--Recipes. 2. Food allergy--Diet therapy--Recipes. I. Bronski, Peter. II. Title.
  RM237.86.B752 2014
  641.5'638--dc23

                              2013037590

ISBN 978-1-61519-100-0
Ebook ISBN 978-1-61519-101-7

Cover design by Susi Oberhelman
Cover photographs by Kelli and Peter Bronski
Author photograph by Kelli and Peter Bronski
Text design by Pauline Neuwirth, Neuwirth & Associates, Inc.

Manufactured in the United States of America

Distributed by Workman Publishing Company, Inc.
Distributed simultaneously in Canada by Thomas Allen & Son Ltd.

First printing June 2014
10 9 8 7 6 5 4 3 2

To our children, Marin, Charlotte, and Timothy

CONTENTS

SIDES AND SNACKS

MAIN MEALS

TASTY TREATS

PREFACE

ANY PARENT IN any household, I think—gluten-free or not—cares about putting delicious, healthy food on the table that kids love to eat. It's part of that innate desire—need, even—to provide for the young persons who are totally dependent upon us. When you introduce a dietary restriction, such as gluten, it only deepens that resolve. It certainly did for us. Doing something for yourself, or even a spouse, is one thing. But there's nothing like the emotion and drive behind doing something for your children.

That part of our story began in late 2008 with the arrival of our first daughter, Marin. She experienced early and seemingly serious digestive issues. To our relief, by the time she turned one, many of those issues had resolved. Later in hindsight, we wondered if perhaps accidental exposure to gluten could have been one of the culprits, though we don't know for certain. But as she migrated to an "adult" diet of all solid foods, there were a handful of instances in which she and I both got sick following the same meals, cases where we suspected gluten cross-contamination was to blame. It appeared Marin was at least as sensitive to gluten as I am, and so we kept her very strictly gluten-free.

That shift to keep her 100 percent gluten-free wasn't much of an adjustment for us. Our household had been gluten-free since early 2007, when I was de facto diagnosed with celiac disease. Kelli voluntarily went gluten-free in the home, too, so that we could enjoy the same, shared meals and also eliminate the possibility that I'd get sick from in-home gluten cross-contamination.

In mid-2010, our second daughter, Charlotte arrived. At the advice of Marin's pediatrician, Kelli had gone completely gluten-free—whether in or outside the home—before the start of her third trimester. Charlotte entered the world a gluten-free child, and we kept her gluten-free proactively out of fear she might be as sensitive as Marin and I were. By the time she was two and a half, she'd never eaten so much as a lick of gluten.

It has been amazing watching our girls in the kitchen, not just observing us, but as eager and active participants. They learned quickly, and that newfound knowledge translated into a different kind of relationship with their food. For example, when visiting grandparents or aunts and uncles, Marin would diligently and confidently ask questions such as: Is this gluten-free? Does this have gluten? It was a matter-of-fact approach, not something that was difficult for either of them to do. They took being gluten-free in stride, perhaps because it is all they had ever known.

They even created fun games of their own about being gluten-free. Playing in the sandbox at a playground, they'd start measuring out different gluten-free flours. Then there was the gluten/gluten-free game they came up with. We'd each take turns being a food at the supermarket. Someone would then ask, "Are you gluten or gluten-free?" If we were gluten, the response would go something along the lines of, "Oh no! You make me sick! My tummy hurts!" And if we were gluten-free, the response would be, "Oh good! I'm going to eat you and gobble you all up! Munch, munch, munch . . ."

Along the way between the arrival of Marin and Charlotte and today, a lot has happened, including the publication of *Artisanal Gluten-Free Cooking* in 2009, *Artisanal Gluten-Free Cupcakes* in 2011, and *Cooking's* revised and updated second edition in 2012. Throughout that time we've received a steady flow of emails from readers who are parents working hard to feed their gluten-free children. Some of those parents have remarked how they've been nearly or literally in tears when their gluten-free child devours a dish prepared from one of our recipes. Few things, if any, are as rewarding for a cookbook author. Helping people is why we write books such as this. Yet scant few cookbooks have specifically focused on gluten-free kids and their families, which is one reason why we felt writing *Gluten-Free Family Favorites* was so important—to provide go-to recipes that would satisfy kids and adults alike, with kid-friendly preparations and flavors compatible with a kid-centric palate.

It's been an interesting time for us, while writing this book. That's because as we finish this manuscript, we've also recently concluded the process of putting Marin and Charlotte through a gluten challenge. They've always been gluten-free, and we'll remain a gluten-free household, but we wanted to know—if at all possible—answers to important questions. How strictly do we need to keep them gluten-free outside the home, such as at school or another person's house, or while traveling, or out to restaurants? Do they have celiac disease or another specific condition that would have implications for their medical care in the coming years? They, and we, needed to know if we could.

We only embarked on that process in early 2013, when Marin was four and Charlotte approaching three, because we wanted to wait until they were old enough to give us specific verbal feedback about how they were feeling during the challenge, which involves eating a minimum "dose" of gluten—via crackers, slices of bread, etc.—for a defined period of time, and then getting a panel of blood tests to check the body's response.

For the girls and us, it was a tough mental shift. Marin and Charlotte had to wrap their heads around eating this thing that had been on the forbidden list for as long as they'd been alive. For Kelli and me, after so carefully avoiding gluten for years, we now had to focus on making sure our girls were eating enough gluten each day to get as reliable test results as we could. Despite how prevalent gluten is in the Standard American Diet, making sure Marin and Charlotte got their requisite "dose" each day was a surprising challenge given that our household is gluten-free. Even figuring out what that dose should be was difficult. Once you've been gluten-free for an extended period of time, the peer-reviewed studies are all over the place on what quantity of daily gluten exposure is appropriate and what duration (one week, two weeks, one month?) yields the most reliable test results, none of which are foolproof. That's one important reason why doctors stress normally getting tested *before* committing to a gluten-free diet.

We expected the worst. Kelli and I both prepared ourselves for the possibility of abandoning the gluten challenge because the girls would get too sick, go through too much pain and discomfort. Yet both girls seemed to handle the gluten well. At least on the surface, nothing—or almost nothing—happened. Marin, whom we suspected to be the more sensitive of the two, had seemingly no problems, including no diarrhea. Charlotte, whom we thought had the "stronger" stomach, also did well but broke out in prominent red rashes over her body.

When the much-anticipated test results came in, both girls tested positive for the celiac disease genes, but negative for celiac disease, at least for now. With their positive genetics and my active symptomology, they're in a higher-risk group. There's no guarantee they'll develop celiac disease, but they could—though celiac disease affects only about one percent of the general population, it's about five times more prevalent among first-degree relatives of someone with the disease.[1] And so we watch and wait. We'll keep an eye out for a change in their health or the emergence of new symptoms that could point to celiac disease, and we'll likely get them retested on some periodic basis to make sure we're not missing anything, such as asymptomatic celiac disease. We're also considering pursuing another round of testing for Charlotte, to explore if a wheat allergy or other condition could be responsible for the rashes she developed.

For now, we're more relaxed with their diet outside the home, though we're trying to keep that outside-the-home gluten consumption to a minimum. Regardless, my own condition remains unchanged and we remain a strictly gluten-free household, which means that all the recipes we make—and all the food we put on the table—needs to satisfy all mouths.

That's our story. But no matter how you've found *Gluten-Free Family Favorites* in your hands—whether you're a gluten-free family, feeding a gluten-free family member or friend, or concerned about the food restrictions of a child's classmate or teammate—this book's recipes can help to feed everyone healthy, delicious gluten-free fare, whether you're all gluten-free or not.

We've included kid-friendly, allergen-friendly, and/or healthier adaptations of some of the popular recipes from our blog, *No Gluten, No Problem,* and our previous cookbooks. We've also added oodles of new recipes that include breakfasts (French toast sticks), snacks (sweet potater tots), dinners (pesto mac and cheese), familiar classics (fish sticks), and tasty treats (waffle cones). Every recipe is of course gluten-free. And as much as possible, we've also included modifications to optionally make recipes free of dairy, eggs, corn, soy, peanuts, tree nuts, and other major allergens, as well as vegetarian and/ or vegan.

So from our gluten-free family to yours, *mangia* and *bon appétit*!

–Peter Bronski, November 2013

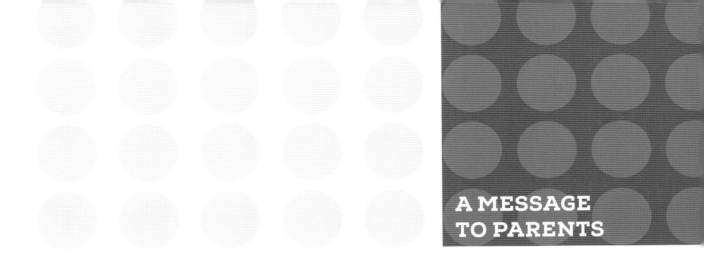

WE HAVE MANY important roles as parents: keeping our children safe yet giving them the freedom to explore and learn from mistakes, nurturing their minds and creativity and innate talents and interests, showing unconditional love and affection while providing structure and discipline. Few roles are as fundamental, though, as feeding them—putting healthy, delicious food on the table that our children love to eat, and that nourishes their bodies and minds so they can grow into the strong, intelligent, vibrant persons you know they can be.

But food and cooking is about much more than offering calories to meet basic biological needs.

For one, it is an opportunity for relationship. It is a chance for you and your child to bond, to reconnect daily in our increasingly busy and scheduled lives. Time spent together as a family in the kitchen preparing a meal, and then eating that meal together around the table, is time very well spent.

Study after study shows that getting kids involved in the kitchen at an early age and eating meals together as a family through adolescence have a multitude of benefits.[2] Children who are engaged with what they eat make healthier dietary choices; are more likely to try new foods; show increased interest in eating fruits and vegetables; become less picky eaters; have decreased rates of obesity; demonstrate higher test scores in school; show fewer signs of depression and stress; and are less likely to engage in smoking, alcohol, and drug use. All that and more from their relationship with family and food.

For kids with food restrictions, gluten-related or otherwise, there are also the critical elements of empowerment and self-confidence. Preparing meals with you makes them more knowledgeable about the foods they eat, the ingredients that go into those foods, and how they're made. That knowledge and the confidence that comes with it can better equip kids to navigate social situations that will inevitably be difficult at times, whether at school, in sports and other extracurricular activities, at parties, or at a friend's house.

It could be that you as the parent are the one who's gluten-free, and that you're bringing your children and household along for the ride, so to speak. But for those parents reading this book who are looking to feed their gluten-free children, how you do or don't embrace the gluten-free "thing" can be critically important for your child.

Consider this real-life example. It was mid-2012, and we were doing a cooking demo and Q&A for a celiac/gluten intolerance support group that met in the community room of a supermarket in north-central New Jersey. There we met two mothers and their daughters who had both been recently diagnosed with celiac disease and were in their first year of college.

One mother was seemingly insensitive and unbending to her daughter's newfound dietary challenges. She told her daughter—and we're paraphrasing only slightly here—"Figure out what you need to do, and when you come home for holidays, make sure you have something you can eat, because we're not changing the way we cook." That's why the mother had brought her daughter to the event. We could see the pain in that daughter's eyes, the way she felt isolated and abandoned at a time when she needed her family's support most.

Then there was the other mother-daughter duo. The mother passionately asked question after question, devouring as much information about gluten-free cooking as she could. Chatting informally after the event, we commended her for taking such steps to safely feed her daughter the kind of food her body needed. The mother went so far as to go gluten-free as well. Her response still rings in our ears word-for-word today: "If it happens to my child, it happens to me."

Though this example involved older children, it nevertheless underscores the centrally important role you play as a parent. You are a role model, a teacher, a guide, a sharer of knowledge and compassion and love. Your children will learn from you. Their relationship with food, health, and their bodies will form in part through your influence and their early formative experiences together with you in the kitchen and at the table.

Make these experiences meaningful and fun. If you're used to running the kitchen, give up some control. Let the kids get their hands (and your kitchen) dirty. Spills, flying flour, knocked-over cups of liquid, a toppled bowl . . . they'll happen; they go with the territory. And don't worry if the recipes don't look photo-ready. The food may look imperfect, but that makes it perfect. A child's experience, confidence, and knowledge come through doing.

The home kitchen and dining room table should be a safe space, one where kids feel they can eat without fear of getting sick, where no food is off-limits, where they don't have to hear the words "No, you can't eat that," where they have positive experiences and build healthy relationships with their bodies and their foods, where they learn that "gluten-free" does in fact set them free, rather than restrict them. You have the power to give them such gifts. Embrace that responsibility and opportunity.

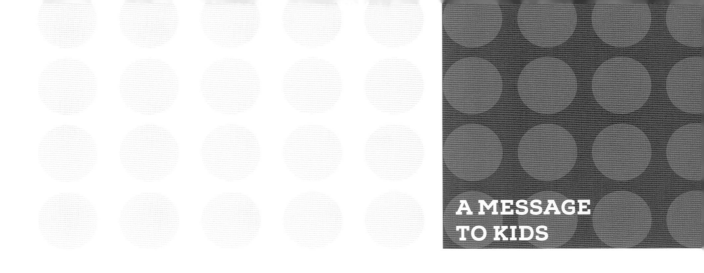

A MESSAGE TO KIDS

PARENTS, WE INVITE you to read this section to the young, gluten-free members of your family.

We hear you're gluten-free. Guess what? We are, too! And so are many people we know, including lots of kids just like you. Some of them have celiac disease. Others have a gluten sensitivity and some have a wheat allergy. This book is for them. And most importantly, this book is for *you*.

We grew up in the kitchen, cooking and baking with our moms and dads and grandmas and grandpas. We made cookies and cakes and breads and pies and lots of other things. It was fun learning how to make all those foods, and it was even more fun to eat them. You can have that kind of fun, too.

We want you to love the food you're eating, and we want you to get your hands messy in the kitchen with your mom or dad making it. Do you know why? Because eating good gluten-free food is the start of something great for you. It's going to help you grow up healthy and strong. It's going to help you feel your best.

We know it can be tough at times. Maybe you're having a snack at school, or a play date at a friend's house, or a dinner with your sports team, or pizza and cake at a birthday party. And sometimes you can't eat those foods that your friends are having. That's happened to us also.

But remember this: Everyone eats different things. Some families are Italian or Chinese, Christian or Jewish, from New York or Georgia or Ohio. People who live in different places, or who come from different places, or who have different families, eat different things. That's one thing that makes food so interesting. There's always something new and tasty to discover.

Being gluten-free is another way to eat that's new and different and very tasty. If you're like us, you eat gluten-free because you need to, because eating foods with gluten will make you sick, and getting sick is no fun. But when the food tastes as good as the recipes you can make in this book, and when that food helps you stay healthy and happy and strong, you'll also hopefully eat gluten-free because you *want* to.

So what are you waiting for? Grab your mom or dad, pick a recipe you want to try, collect your ingredients, and get in the kitchen and start cooking! You can make yummy gluten-free food, just like us and lots of gluten-free kids just like you!

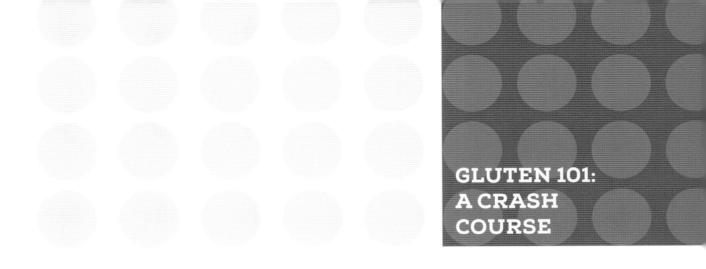

IF YOU'RE GOING to foster a happy, healthy, and well-fed gluten-free family and household, you need to first understand what gluten is and where to find it. In this instance, it pays to follow the advice of ancient Chinese military general and philosopher Sun Tzu, who challenged us in his classic *The Art of War* to both "know yourself" *and* "know your enemy." Not that this is a true battle, but we *are* drawing some pretty important lines in the kitchen.

What is gluten?

When we talk about *gluten,* we're specifically referring to the family of storage proteins found in wheat, barley, and rye and their relatives and crossbreeds that cause problems for people with gluten intolerance (celiac disease, gluten sensitivity, wheat allergy, etc.). Wheat and its proteins glutenin and gliadin are by far the most common offenders, though *wheat-free* and *gluten-free* are not exactly the same thing. A product could be wheat-free but still have gluten from rye and especially barley, which is a common ingredient in breakfast cereals and other foods such as some teas, some soups, malt vinegar, and beer.

Grains to avoid

These grains contain gluten (or, in the case of oats, are liable to cross-contamination):

Wheat	Spelt*
Barley	Durum
Rye	Semolina
Einkorn	Triticale
Emmer	Oats (if not certified gluten-free)

*If you dig around the Internet, you're likely to come across claims that ancient varieties of wheat such as spelt are gluten-free. They are *not*.

Foods to avoid

You'll want to avoid foods traditionally made from the flours of gluten-containing grains:

Bagels	Noodles (e.g., udon)
Bread	Pancakes
Breakfast cereals	Pasta (including couscous)
Bulgur	Pies
Cakes	Pizza
Cookies	Waffles
Farina	

Other names for gluten

When you're reading ingredients labels, gluten isn't always screaming at you in big, bold letters, though allergen and gluten-free labeling standards (see page 9) are helping with that. Be watchful for the following terms, which indicate the presence of gluten:

Barley malt	Modified food starch (especially if the source isn't identified)
Hydrolyzed wheat gluten	
Malt	Wheat gluten
Malt flavoring	

Places where gluten can hide

In addition to the usual suspects, gluten can hide in a number of places, including but not limited to:

Canned soups	Sauces and marinades
Imitation crabmeat	Seitan
Processed meats	Soy sauce

Cross-contamination concerns

Serving gluten-free food is about two things: 1) reliably gluten-free ingredients, and 2) the safe preparation and handling of gluten-free foods.

Cross-contamination is when food that is ordinarily gluten-free picks up gluten from other foods or by way of utensils or equipment in the manufacturing facility or kitchen.

Remember that for a highly sensitive individual with a condition such as celiac disease, it takes very little gluten to cause damage, whether that person experiences obvious and immediate symptoms or not. Ensuring gluten-free ingredients is relatively straightforward (see page 9 for more details); nevertheless, it pays to remain vigilant. That's especially true when it comes to the preparation and handling of gluten-free foods, particularly if you have a shared kitchen (not to mention circumstances where you're dining out at a restaurant, having a meal at a relative or friend's house, or attending a school party, sports team meal, or play date).

It's not enough for meals to be made of gluten-free ingredients. The integrity of their gluten-free status must be maintained from pantry to plate (and everywhere in between).

10 TIPS FOR AVOIDING CROSS-CONTAMINATION

IF YOU'RE ABLE to establish an entirely gluten-free kitchen, avoiding cross-contamination becomes much simpler and life that much easier for the gluten-free members of your family. But if you have both gluten-free and non-gluten-free items in your pantry and kitchen, by following these tips and using regular vigilance, you can still ensure that the gluten-free people at your table can safely enjoy gluten-free meals.

1. Purge your pantry of non-gluten-free items (best option) or store items in a way that maintains strict separation of gluten-free and non-gluten-free items (e.g., keep gluten-free flour in its own, airtight container).

2. Wash dishes, utensils, and other implements in a dishwasher. Also thoroughly wash pots, pans, work surfaces, etc.—ideally with a new sponge if your old sponge has been around the gluten block for a while. (Better yet, have two sponges: one for gluten-free items and the other for non-gluten-free items.)

3. Use a dedicated cutting board and knife (best option) or be sure to slice gluten-free items first before handling any non-gluten-free items, then thoroughly wash everything when you're done.

4. No double dipping! Prominently label items such as jelly and peanut butter with a permanent marker or "GF" sticker and make them dedicated gluten-free (best option) or be super-vigilant to avoid double dipping, such as after you've already spread butter, jelly, or whatever on a slice of wheat toast.

5. No sharing! You may teach your kids to share their toys, but when it comes to food preparation and serving, there's no sharing here. If you have both gluten-free and non-gluten-free items on the table, each

(continued)

gets its own serving spoon. Ditto for spatulas if you're flipping gluten-free and regular pancakes on two griddles.

6. Be water wise. In the famous children's book *Strega Nona*, the grandma witch boiled up some pasta nice and hot in her magical pasta pot. At your home, make sure the gluten-free pasta cooks in its own special pot and doesn't mingle with "regular" pasta water.

7. Beware of crumbs! If you can assign a toaster oven or toaster to be exclusively gluten-free, great! But if you must share one appliance, be careful to avoid getting gluten crumbs on gluten-free toast and other items—try using a sheet of foil in a toaster oven or a toaster bag (a specialty product that prevents gluten crumbs in a toaster from ever coming into contact with your gluten-free bread) in a conventional stand-up toaster.

8. Assign a gluten-free prep zone in your kitchen where only gluten-free foods are handled (no tossing wheat flour for a pizza dough next to the gluten-free pizza!).

9. Educate! Guidelines such as these don't do any good if people don't know about them or follow them. Make sure everyone in your family—and your kitchen—knows the rules of the gluten-free road.

10. Adjust accordingly. We all have different levels of sensitivity. For some people, steps such as these will be more than sufficient. For others, nothing short of an entire dedicated gluten-free kitchen will do. Take the steps you and your body need to safely eat gluten-free. Your health is worth it.

ACCORDING TO THE Food Marketing Institute, the average supermarket in 2010 (the most recent year for which data is available) carried nearly 39,000 products.[3] A growing number of those products are for the gluten-free community.

The research firm Packaged Facts predicts the gluten-free market will exceed $6 billion by 2017,[4] with a compound annual growth rate of 28 percent between 2008 and 2012.[5] And the research firm Mintel already put the market past $6 billion in 2011.[6]

No matter how you slice it, the gluten-free market is growing, and fast. But with such growth and a seemingly ever-expanding number of options at the supermarket, how to know what is and isn't safe? It's time to become a savvy supermarket shopper.

Always read labels

Naturally gluten-free foods—such as the fresh fruits and vegetables of the produce section—obviously don't have a label. But there's a maxim many follow in the gluten-free community: if it has an ingredient label, read the label. Every time. You'd be surprised how many places gluten can hide. Even products that have been gluten-free in the past may not be now, since product formulations and manufacturing facilities can change.

There are a number of smartphone apps (such as the Is That Gluten Free? app) and printed guides (such as Triumph Dining's *The Essential Gluten-Free Grocery Guide*) designed to help you navigate the potential minefield of what is and isn't safely gluten-free in the supermarket. But your best bet is to become an educated and religiously committed label reader. Despite best attempts to update content, third-party information from apps and guides can go out of date. You're better off checking the product labels because, in theory, the packaging should always accurately reflect its ingredients.

Allergen labeling

Thanks to the United States' Food Allergen Labeling and Consumer Protection Act of 2004 (FALCPA), manufacturers are required to declare when a product contains one of the top eight most common food allergens: milk, eggs, fish, shellfish, tree nuts, peanuts, wheat, and soy.[7] Such declarations must take one or both of two forms:

1. If the ingredients list doesn't clearly state the common name of an allergen, it must parenthetically note the allergen—e.g., "flour (wheat)."
2. Immediately after or next to the regular ingredients list it must include a "contains" statement—e.g., "contains wheat."

Advisory labeling

In addition to mandatory allergen labeling, manufacturers can voluntarily declare what *may* be in their product due to potential cross-contamination, such as from a shared production line. This is known as advisory labeling.[8] Such label statements will usually take the form of either "may contain wheat" or "processed in a facility (or on machinery) that also processes wheat." Depending on your level of sensitivity and acceptable risk, advisory labeling can be a major red flag, no big deal, or somewhere in between.

Gluten-free labeling

In August 2013, the U.S. Food and Drug Administration (FDA) released the ruling on its long-awaited gluten-free labeling standard.[9] There is now clear guidance on when and how companies may make a "gluten-free" claim about their product and on its packaging. The standard boils down to a single number: 20 parts per million (ppm). That's the threshold for gluten content at which a company can no longer make the gluten-free claim about a product. It applies whether a food is inherently gluten-free or contains wheat, barley, rye, or their direct relatives or crossbreeds that has been processed to remove the gluten. The 20 ppm number aligns with the Codex Alimentarius, the international standard[10]—scientific consensus confirms that 20 ppm is within safe limits for people with celiac disease, though some in the gluten-free community maintain that more stringent (even zero tolerance) standards should be in place. The FDA ruling applies to restaurants as well as food companies. But keep in mind that gluten-free claims on packaging or menus are voluntary. Don't restrict your choices to only those foods and products that are explicitly labeled as gluten-free; a world of options beyond such labeled foods is open to you.

Independent third-party certification

In addition to the federal gluten-free labeling standard, consumers can seek added peace of mind through products certified by independent third-party programs. For example, one popular program is the Gluten-Free Certification Organization (GFCO) of the Gluten Intolerance Group. It claims to have certified some 13,000 gluten-free products as of February 2013 and fully one quarter of the gluten-free product market during 2012. Another is the Gluten-Free Certification Program (GFCP), a joint effort of the US-based National Foundation for Celiac Awareness and the Canadian Celiac Association, announced in 2013. Both the GFCO and GFCP certify products at a gluten limit of 10 ppm, twice as stringent as the FDA standard.

---

3 ESSENTIAL TIPS FOR BEING A SAVVY SUPERMARKET SHOPPER

1. Focus your grocery shopping on the perimeter of the supermarket, where you'll find naturally gluten-free whole foods such as fresh fruits and vegetables, nuts and seeds, legumes, whole meats and fish, eggs, and dairy (including milk, butter, cheese, and yogurt).
2. Religiously read the ingredients on any food or product that has a label. (But you knew that already now, didn't you?)
3. Beware bulk bins, which can pose a serious cross-contamination risk. For example, maybe someone used the same scoop in both gluten-free rice and glutenous bulgur.

Also be sure to check out the Money Matters section (page 14) for a number of tips on reducing your family's gluten-free grocery bill.

FOOD AND KITCHEN SAFETY

COOKING WITH KIDS is fun and rewarding, but the kitchen can also be a dangerous place if you're not careful. Crosby, Stills, Nash, and Young sang to "teach your children well." We should do that and more, building sound skills and good habits. If we do, our children can enjoy safe times in the kitchen cooking with us, and look forward to a lifetime of memories, skills, and benefits that go along with it.

Adult supervision

Supervise your children when they are cooking in the kitchen with you. You are teaching skills that will eventually enable their self-sufficiency, but you must also be their guide, role model, and safety enforcer. Sometimes children can and need to directly experience negative outcomes and receive visceral feedback, but the kitchen is rarely the place for it. The consequences of a bad burn or cut, for example, can be too severe.

Also, we've said it elsewhere but it bears repeating here. Though we make suggestions for ways to get kids involved in the preparation of each recipe, you as their parent must assign tasks that are age and ability appropriate.

Washing hands

Children should learn to wash their hands before handling food, as well as after any times they've been exposed to germs—blowing their nose, touching raw meat, etc.

Knives

You've probably heard the phrase "a safe knife is a sharp knife." That's true, but when it comes to the youngest members of your family, sometimes the safest knife is no knife at all. When you do introduce knives, teach your children good technique early—how to hold the knife, the food, the hand and fingers, how to cut away from the body. Start them with foods that can be cut with a butter knife, such as mushrooms, tofu, the flesh of an avocado, or the red part of a watermelon, so that they can practice and develop the fine motor skills to eventually become confident with a "real" knife.

Feeling hot, hot, hot

Have your children be extra careful around hot stoves, ovens, pots, and pans. We don't want any bad burns! Be similarly careful around boiling water (212°F/100°C at sea level) and steam (which can get much hotter).

Power tools

Some recipes might involve using the kitchen equivalent of power tools: blenders, food processors, immersion blenders, electric beaters, stand-up electric mixers. They have fast-moving parts with powerful motors, and sometimes, sharp blades. Though some, such as a food processor, typically have one or more safety mechanisms that prevent them from being turned on without protective measures in place (such as the lid), make sure to teach your children that hands never go in or near them, whether they're actually turned on or not.

Making tasks younger-kid-accessible

You have a variety of options for how your younger kids can engage with recipe tasks: bring them up onto the kitchen countertop (requires very close supervision), put them on stools or stable chairs so they can reach, and move tasks to the kitchen table or a low kids' table rather than the counter, for example. It's all about making the food safely accessible and within your and your kids' comfort zone. Our younger daughter, Charlotte, once fell off the counter, hit her chin on the floor, and nearly bit clean through her tongue. Sorry for the graphic imagery, but it's an important cautionary tale. Cooking with your children should end with a delicious shared meal, not a trip to the emergency room.

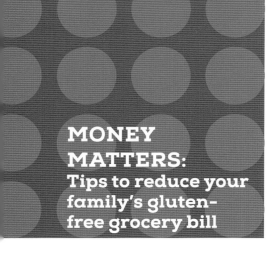

MONEY MATTERS:
Tips to reduce your family's gluten-free grocery bill

FEEDING A FAMILY isn't cheap these days. According to the USDA's Center for Nutrition Policy and Promotion, in 2013 the average American family of four with school-age children on a moderate budget spent more than $238 per week on groceries, or almost $12,400 per year, assuming all meals were prepared and eaten at home.[11]

The burden can be even greater on gluten-free families. A series of studies published between 2007 and 2011 in publications such as the *Journal of Human Nutrition and Dietetics* and *Canadian Journal of Dietetic Practice and Research* found that gluten-free products and the gluten-free diet can be anywhere from 76 to 500-plus percent more expensive than their standard, wheat-based counterparts.[12] That's a hefty premium.

But a healthy, gluten-free diet with meals your kids love doesn't have to break the bank. Follow these tips to reduce your family's gluten-free grocery bill:

1. *Focus on naturally gluten-free, whole foods.*

    You've heard this before: the foundation of a sound gluten-free diet should find you frequenting the periphery of your supermarket . . . and perhaps your garden, a local farmers' market, CSA share, you name it. That's where you'll find whole meats and fish, yogurt, milk, cheese, eggs, fresh fruits and vegetables, legumes, nuts and seeds, and gluten-free grains (such as rice, corn, quinoa, buckwheat, sorghum, teff, and millet). These form the basis of a deliciously healthy gluten-free diet. And here's the bonus: because they're naturally gluten-free and just plain good food, they cost the same whether you're gluten-free or not. Zero premium. Zip. Zilch. Nada. A chicken is a chicken; an apple is an apple. Certified gluten-free versions of naturally gluten-free grains, however, can cost more.

2. *Eat fewer gluten-free specialty foods.*

Remember those staggering statistics we just cited, about how gluten-free products can cost upwards of *500-plus percent* more than their standard, wheat-based counterparts? Well, that applies primarily to store-bought, gluten-free versions of specialty foods: breads, pizza crusts, cereals, cookies, crackers, pasta, baking mixes, etc. In early 2013 our own conservative estimate, published on *No Gluten, No Problem*, of what this "gluten-free premium" adds up to annually was nearly $800.[13] That's no small piece of pocket change, and the number could easily be higher. The solution: eat fewer of those price-inflated, specialty gluten-free foods. It's as simple as that.

3. *Make your baked goods from scratch.*

We're not saying you should completely do without. It's great to have a sandwich on good gluten-free bread, a hot pizza for dinner, or the occasional cookie. But you can be kinder to your bank account by making many of these items yourself from scratch. (You're holding this cookbook in your hands, so hopefully you're going down that road already!) Take our Artisan Gluten-Free Flour Blend (page 27) and recipes for bread, pizza dough, and cookies as examples. We ran the numbers (again for *No Gluten, No Problem* in 2013) and confirmed that from-scratch baking is often the way to go.[14] For example, most all-purpose, gluten-free flour blends sell for $4 to almost $7 per pound; our flour blend—mixed from scratch using component ingredients purchased at our local supermarket—cost $2.27 per pound. Bingo. The story was the same for the bread, pizza dough, and cookies: you pay anywhere from 66 to 150 percent *more* to buy gluten-free versions at the store.

4. *Take the gluten-free tax deduction.*

Despite your best attempts to minimize your gluten-free grocery bill, there's still a good chance that you'll pay more at the cash register than you would if you were on the Standard American Diet. For some families, those extra costs may add up enough to make taking a deduction on your annual federal income tax both possible and worthwhile.[15] Mind you, taking that deduction comes with a number of caveats: you must be gluten-free for a medically diagnosed reason (such as celiac disease, wheat allergy, or non-celiac gluten sensitivity) with a doctor's note, you must keep all receipts and religiously track the premium you pay to maintain your gluten-free diet, and the gluten-free premium—when added to other qualifying medical expenses—must exceed 10 percent of your adjusted gross income. Organizations such as the National Foundation for Celiac Awareness, Celiac Disease

Foundation, Celiac Support Association, and Kogan Celiac Center offer excellent resources on the tax write-off (see page 198 for information on these resources). And of course, we'd be remiss if we didn't suggest you consult a tax professional on the details and potential implications of taking the deduction.

5. ## *Budget and track expenses.*

   Whether you take the gluten-free tax deduction or not, set a weekly family grocery budget, keep your receipts, and track your food costs over time. Simply staying aware of your expenses helps to keep them in check. You're much less likely to blow your budget or make impulse purchases.

6. ## *Plan your meals each week.*

   According to a 2012 study from the Natural Resources Defense Council, Americans throw away roughly 40 percent (!) of their food each year.[16] The NRDC study estimated all that wasted food totaled $165 billion annually, or $2,275 per year for the average American family of four. Hello, money-saving opportunity! Planning your meals for the week, and then aligning your weekly grocery shopping to buy mostly what you'll need for those meals specifically (rather than wandering the supermarket aimlessly for random foods), will drastically reduce the amount of food—and money—you throw away.

7. ## *Stock up during sales.*

   Thrifty shoppers know how to capture maximum value from sales. Part of that strategy includes brand flexibility, buying whatever brand of a given food happens to be on sale in any particular week. As gluten-free consumers, we don't have the luxury. When we find a gluten-free company that we know, love, and trust, we tend to remain fiercely loyal. Besides, gluten-free foods don't tend to go on sale all that often anyway. (When's the last time you saw your favorite gluten-free pasta on a super saver special?) Fortunately, though, staple foods *do* often go on sale— butter, rice, olive oil, chicken. And when they do, stock up! Store them in your pantry or freezer, and plan to use them over the coming weeks or even months.

8. ## *Make creative use of leftovers.*

   And speaking of reducing food waste, don't you dare send those leftovers to the garbage, at least not yet! (Unless they're moldy or otherwise not edible. . . . In that case, by all means get them out of the kitchen, preferably as compost.) Instead, make creative use of leftovers to help your food go further. Loaf of bread starting to go stale? Transform it into good-as-new French toast sticks and enjoy it for breakfast. Or turn it into bread crumbs for meatballs, chicken fingers, or fish sticks. Didn't finish last night's steak? Give it new life in a gluten-free beef stroganoff.

9. *Eat more veggies and less meat.*

Back in the mid-twentieth century, when our grandparents were busy raising our parents, meat was a relative delicacy—expensive, and eaten in smaller quantities a handful of times each week. The wisdom then was that if you wanted to save money on your food, an easy place to do it was with meat. Cut back your consumption in favor of more vegetables, and you'd notice the financial difference. For a multitude of reasons, meat has become much cheaper, and as a result we're eating a lot more of it. According to the Earth Policy Institute and the USDA, throughout the first half of the twentieth century, American per capita annual meat consumption hovered around 100 pounds; for the last few decades, it's been over 160 pounds (and as high as 195).[17] Even so, there's still a good chance that by swapping out some of your meat-based weekly meals for vegetarian ones you can cut back on your grocery bill.

10. *Incorporate less expensive cuts of meat.*

You're probably not having filet mignon every night for dinner. (We certainly aren't!) After all, it's expensive. Yet we Americans love certain premium cuts of meat. Take the ubiquitous boneless, skinless—and relatively pricey—chicken breast. It's the most desirable part of the bird, and whether you realize it or not, we pay to be able to buy it trimmed and ready for cooking. According to a 2012 consumer survey by the National Chicken Council, 85 percent of consumers buy boneless, skinless chicken breasts either regularly or when they're on sale.[18] Meanwhile, only 9 percent of consumers buy such chicken breasts rarely, if ever, in favor of less expensive legs, thighs, or the whole chicken. Yet that's a great opportunity. Use cheaper thighs to make chicken teriyaki, or cook a whole chicken, which can be roasted and then the carcass used to make stock, or quartered raw and simmered to make homemade chicken soup.

11. *Splurge strategically.*

If you're like us, in a perfect world you'd buy all organic produce and all ethical/humane meats all the time. Sadly, such choices too often add expense to your grocery bill. Sure, we'd like to do all our shopping at the equivalent of a Whole Foods, but that's simply not in the cards. Like most American families, we're on a budget, making the best decisions we can for our family within the realistic bounds of our finances. That's why it pays, literally, to splurge strategically. For example, use a resource such as the Environmental Working Group's annual *Shopper's Guide to Pesticides in Produce* (available for free on its website, ewg.org) to inform your choices.[19] The guide's Dirty Dozen Plus and Clean Fifteen lists highlight the most- and least-contaminated fruits and vegetables. Concentrate on buying organic for the worst offenders, and give your wallet a break on the rest.

12. **Eat less. Seriously.**

As a cost-cutting measure, eating less may sound either ridiculously obvious or obviously ridiculous, but hear us out. First, if you or a member of your family is regaining his or her health on a gluten-free diet after suffering the effects of a condition such as celiac disease, then that healing will likely come with increased intestinal nutrient absorption. In other words, you'll benefit from a greater percentage of the food you're eating—rather than it going straight through you—and so may need to downsize portions as a result. Second, depending on the makeup of your diet to date, it may be time to focus more on nutrient-dense whole foods (see tip #1). According to the *Journal of Nutrition*, empty-calorie foods with excessive sugar and fat taste great in the moment and are relatively cheap, but they come with costs: They lack the nutrients we need, they don't satisfy our hunger, and we eat them in much larger portions, which can offset their initially cheaper sticker price.[20] Finally, according to the "Profiling Food Consumption in America" chapter of the USDA's *Agriculture Fact Book*, Americans' average daily calorie intake increased by nearly 25 percent between 1970 and 2000 alone.[21] We're likely eating far more calories than we need. Eat less.

13. **Skip the restaurants and dine in.**

Who doesn't love to go out to eat every now and then? We sure do! But as a 2011 *Time* magazine article showed, dining out at restaurants—even for so-called cheap fast food—quickly becomes more expensive than a healthy home-cooked meal.[22] Yet Americans love to dine out. Survey after survey shows that we eat out an incredible four to five times per week, or 200 to 250 restaurant meals per year.[23] But despite restaurant meals making up some 25 percent of our weekly meals, they account for 47 percent of our food dollars, according to 2013 statistics from the National Restaurant Association.[24] That's consistent with stats from the U.S. Bureau of Labor Statistics for 2011—the most recent year for which full federal data is available—that similarly showed Americans spend more than 40 percent of our food dollars on meals away from home.[25] And while the gluten-free community has somewhat shied away from restaurants in the past, as more and more restaurants accommodate gluten-free diners, we're dining out more, too. For example, gluten-free takeout orders on GrubHub increased by 60 percent between April 2012 and mid-2013.[26] Unfortunately, we're paying for it. Not only do restaurant meals cost more than meals prepared at home, but in the majority of cases, restaurants add a surcharge for gluten-free versions of regular menu items, such as when substituting gluten-free pasta, bread, or pizza crust.

14. *Be a savvy shopper.*

You may not have noticed this, but sometimes it can be hard to find your favorite gluten-free products—or *any* gluten-free products—in certain stores or regions of the country. With the recent explosive growth in popularity of and demand for gluten-free foods, availability is rapidly on the rise. But for now, availability remains widely varied. For example, a pair of studies from 2007 and 2011 issues of the *Journal of Human Nutrition and Dietetics* found that the availability of gluten-free products ranged from almost non-existent to virtually guaranteed as you went from convenience stores to budget supermarkets and independent grocery stores to regular chain supermarkets to upscale supermarkets to health food stores to the Internet.[27] Meanwhile, a series of studies from the *Journal of Consumer Affairs, Preventive Medicine,* and the *Journal of the American Dietetic Association* found that the prices for a given food varied widely from store type to store type.[28] Do your research and figure out where you can get which gluten-free foods at what prices. In these cases, a little bit of effort can go a long way, such as when we discovered xanthan gum from Bob's Red Mill for $5 at one store (sadly, only a temporary price drop), compared to a whopping $12 everywhere else.

15. *Time is money.*

Families can get busy. Between work, school, extracurricular activities, and other demands, time is precious. So make your time in the kitchen count. Whether dinner rolls, chocolate chip cookies, or meatballs, make larger batches, then portion them off and freeze for easy later use. You'll free up more of your time for other activities, and when the refrigerator and/or pantry are looking empty and you're feeling tempted to go out to eat, you'll have tasty gluten-free meals ready to eat with a simple defrost and reheat.

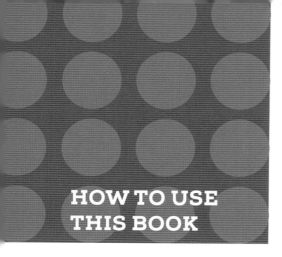

HOW TO USE THIS BOOK

BEFORE WE GET started cooking, here are a few notes about how we've structured the recipes that'll be helpful for you to know. Every recipe follows a similar format: name, yield, headnote, ingredients, steps, allergen-friendly modifications, kid involvement. Here are a few things to keep in mind about specific items:

Yield

An indication of how much food the recipe makes. If a recipe makes units of food—numbers of muffins or cookies or meatballs, for instance—we give you that number. For other recipes, we've tried to give an indication of the number of servings the recipe yields, assuming two adults and the remainder young children. For example, if a recipe makes six servings, it'd feed roughly two adults and four young children. But if you have adolescents with voracious appetites, you should treat them as adults and adjust the recipe's yield accordingly. That recipe that says it feeds six might only feed four in your case. Such are the challenges of defining a serving size when the mouths you're feeding could range from a toddler to a teen.

Ingredients

Not much to say about this except that in cases where you should pay extra attention to the gluten-free status of an ingredient, we've called it out by noting "GF" in front of the ingredient name. For example, most soy sauce contains wheat, so we indicate "GF tamari wheat-free soy sauce or GF soy sauce." Of course, there are always surprises, so we recommend you check *every* label.

Allergen-friendly modifications

This is where you'll find specific instructions for how to make a variation of the recipe that avoids specific allergens but doesn't sacrifice taste. Every recipe in this book is gluten-free, but we've also endeavored to make the recipes as accessible as possible to other dietary restrictions, and be ridiculously transparent about that information. We've included the Top 8 allergens, plus other restrictions frequently associated with those who are gluten-free, and other common dietary choices:

Peanuts	Dairy/lactose/casein
Tree nuts	Corn
Soy	Refined sugar
Fish	Vegetarian
Shellfish	Vegan
Eggs	Grains

Kids can . . .

Although you could just make any of the recipes in this book yourself, the intention is for your children to help you prepare the meals, and in this section we highlight suggestions for ways to get them involved. Of course, you know your kids a whole lot better than we do, so supervise and assign them tasks that are age and skill appropriate as you see fit. And if you haven't already, read the Food and Kitchen Safety section (page 12) as well. Please.

A note about ingredients

Throughout this book our recipes call for familiar ingredients you're likely to find in your kitchen at home, or that you'd easily be able to find at many supermarkets. Here are a few things to keep in mind about particular items:

Butter – We use salted butter at home for flavor, but if sodium consumption is a concern, by all means use unsalted butter. We simply specify "butter" in recipes so you can decide.

Eggs – When we call for eggs, by default we mean large eggs (about 57 g, including shell). If you want to make an egg-free version of a baked good, substitute 1 tablespoon ground flaxseeds and 3 tablespoons warm water *per egg*. Allow the mixture to set for at least 2 minutes before using. Don't worry about doing the calculations—we give specific amounts with each recipe.

Milk – When we call for milk, we mean dairy or cow's milk. The most popular in our home is 2%, though feel free to use skim (nonfat), 1%, or whole milk. We also give instructions throughout for substituting non-dairy milks, such as almond, soy, rice, or hemp. Some recipes call for milk powder, which is also referred to as powdered milk or dry milk. It's simply milk that has been dehydrated, and it can typically be found in the canned milk section of supermarkets.

Oats – Some recipes call for oats. Make sure you're using certified gluten-free oats. They're more expensive, but it's an important distinction. Non-certified oats are often cross-contaminated with gluten and not safe if you have celiac disease or another sensitive condition.

Olive oil – Throughout this cookbook, when we call for olive oil we mean extra light olive oil. It's not the same as extra virgin olive oil, so please take note. Extra light olive oil has a lighter flavor and a higher smoke point, making it a better choice for sautéing and other uses in our recipes.

Sugar – When a recipe calls for sugar, we mean white, granulated sugar. If a recipe calls for more than one type of sugar, then we'll specify granulated sugar. Throughout the book you'll also find other sweeteners, including light and dark brown sugar (if we don't specify light or dark, use either), honey, and agave nectar. When possible, we've given modifications to make refined-sugar-free versions of recipes, though not often for desserts. A little sugar in moderation for dessert is okay with us. For classification purposes, we consider granulated sugar, light brown sugar, and dark brown sugar to be refined, and coconut sugar, honey, agave nectar, and maple syrup to be not.

Yeast – Some recipes, especially breads and our pizza dough, call for yeast. By default we mean active dry yeast, which can be bought either in packets or in small jars.

US vs. metric measurements

Throughout this cookbook, you'll find a recipe's ingredients list expressed in both United States and metric measurements. Here are some guidelines to keep in mind:

1. If we call for an ingredient by unit (e.g., 2 large chicken breasts, 3 medium onions), we leave the unit. An onion is an onion, whether you're in the US or not.

2. If we call for a liquid ingredient by volume, we include both US cups (and/or fluid ounces) *and* milliliters. One common US cup equals approximately 237 ml, which we round to 240 ml (vs. 250 ml for a metric cup).

3. If we call for an ingredient by tablespoon or teaspoon, we list only that measurement, since US and European metric tablespoons and teaspoons are more or less identical.

4. If we call for an ingredient by weight, we include both ounces/ pounds *and* grams/kilograms.

5. If we call for an ingredient by volume of more than ¼ cup (e.g., 1 cup flour, ½ cup diced onion, ¾ cup chopped cilantro), we also list its weight in grams.

A note about canned ingredients: Most canned goods in the United States are sold in cans ranging from 13.5 ounces (383 g) to 15 ounces (425 g). Most European canned goods are sold in 400 g cans. If one of our recipes calls for an entire can of an ingredient, we've listed both its US ounce size and its specific metric equivalent, but feel free to simply substitute one whole 400 g can for convenience.

A note about metric conversions: When we've calculated the metric weight of an ingredient, we've done so with accuracy to the single gram. Feel free, however, to round to the nearest 5 grams, depending on the accuracy of your scale and/or convenience. For convenient volume measuring, we have already rounded to the nearest 5 milliliters.

Convenience shortcuts

As you'll see, we're big fans of from-scratch cooking and baking. But we can appreciate the time-saving convenience of shortcuts as much as the next busy family. So when you're in a pinch, remember that a well-chosen store-bought item can simplify things. Sure, we include a recipe for Smoky Tomato Salsa on page 107, but that doesn't mean you can't substitute your favorite jarred or fresh salsa from the store. Ditto for the recipe for a simple, home-made marinara sauce that accompanies the Spaghetti Squash "Pasta" on page 92. We're not ashamed to admit we keep a jar of quality marinara sauce in the pantry for nights when we want the easy, quick, convenient option. Always remember: while we often empower you to make delicious gluten-free meals from scratch, you can embrace that "from-scratch" ethic as much—or as little—as you'd like.

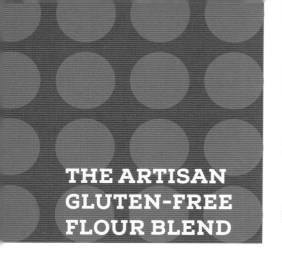

THE ARTISAN GLUTEN-FREE FLOUR BLEND

ONE SECRET TO great gluten-free baking is a great all-purpose gluten-free flour blend. But which blend to use? With more than a dozen blends available ready-made at stores and over the Internet, and scores more available as mix-your-own blend recipes in cookbooks and on blogs, the sheer number of options can feel paralyzing. Here's a quick-and-dirty primer on what you need to know.

A world of flours

Though losing the kitchen staple of inexpensive and ubiquitous wheat flour can initially feel restrictive, think about this: you've lost one flour, but your world of baking has been opened to many more! Options include grains (brown rice, sorghum, millet, buckwheat, quinoa, teff, corn), nuts (almond, coconut, hazelnut), legumes (garbanzo bean, fava bean, soy, green pea, lentil), and starchy roots and fruits (potato, tapioca, arrowroot, banana). No single gluten-free flour tends to be the perfect substitute for wheat, so a blend that combines flours usually works best.

"Faking" the gluten

No matter what combination of flours you use to make a gluten-free blend, they all share one thing in common: they lack gluten. But the gluten, of course, is what makes baked goods "do their thing." It enables doughs and batters to maintain their structure and hold their rise during baking. Gluten-free flours typically "fake" the gluten with the addition of either xanthan gum, guar gum, flax gel, or psyllium husks to mimic the role gluten would otherwise play.

The convenience factor

Some approaches to gluten-free baking require you to keep myriad individual flours on hand, and to mix them in varying ratios on a recipe-by-recipe basis. Our approach, on the other hand, has been to develop a single all-purpose blend that you can mix in however large or small a quantity as you like, and use it in *every* recipe with stellar results. Having the mix on-hand introduces a major convenience factor, an important consideration when working to feed a busy family. And as an added bonus, a great all-purpose blend—like ours—can typically also be substituted cup for cup when converting other wheat-flour-based recipes to gluten-free status.

Nutrition

Some starches in a gluten-free flour blend do wonders for the texture of your baked goods, but too much starch causes you to sacrifice nutrition. Your baked goods can end up filled with too many empty carb calories and not much else. On the other hand, nut, legume, and whole grain flours can boost the protein, fiber, and other nutrition content of your blend. For example, one comparison we did of a dozen all-purpose blends found that nutrition-rich blends had *triple* the protein content of starch-based blends.[29]

The making of our blend

We spent what felt like ages developing the recipe for our Artisan Gluten-Free Flour Blend. Imagine spending months and months baking batch after batch of cookies, pancakes, and more, using various versions of a flour blend with different ratios and ingredients. (That was us, circa 2008.) The result was what we think is one of the best all-purpose gluten-free flour blends you'll ever use, and it's been the basis for every baking recipe we've subsequently developed for our blog, *No Gluten, No Problem,* and our cookbooks, including *Artisanal Gluten-Free Cooking, Artisanal Gluten-Free Cupcakes,* and this book. In recipes, you'll see it referenced as "Artisan GF Flour Blend" for short. It combines "whole" flours that boost its protein and fiber with starches that yield exceptional texture in the finished food.

Here are a few things to keep in mind when making the blend:

Accurately measuring flour

There are two primary ways to measure flour in a recipe: by weight or by volume. Measuring by weight is by far the more accurate measure. Volumetric measuring depends on how tightly you pack the flour into your measuring cup. In one test we performed, we found that the weight of a cup of flour could vary by as much as *44 percent!*

If you're going to measure by volume, follow these simple instructions for the most accurate results every time: First use a spoon to stir and lightly aerate your master batch of flour. Then spoon the flour from your master batch into your measuring cup, without packing down the flour at all. Finally, use a straight edge such as a knife to level the measured cup of flour.

If you're going to measure by weight, digital scales are an inexpensive and very worthwhile addition to your kitchen. Look for a model that registers weight in single-gram increments (some scales measure 5 g at a time) and that has a 10-pound or so max capacity (some scales max out at much lower weights, which limits how big a bowl you can use and how much flour you can mix at once). With a scale, mixing up a batch of flour is super convenient: Set a large bowl on the scale and press the "tare" button to zero the scale. Add the first ingredient until you reach the desired weight, tare the scale again, add the second ingredient until you reach its desired weight, and so on until you've added all the ingredients and are ready to mix.

Ingredient substitutions

If you have a dietary sensitivity to a component of our flour blend, don't worry. Try these ingredient substitutions to mix an alternate version that will meet your dietary needs and still yield similar results:

Corn – Omit the cornstarch and replace with arrowroot flour (a shy ½ cup for a single batch, 1¾ cups for a quadruple batch).

Potato – Omit the potato starch and potato flour and replace with tapioca starch (⅓ cup total for a single batch, 1⅓ cups total for a quadruple batch).

Sorghum – Omit the sorghum and replace with additional brown rice flour.

Xanthan gum – Xanthan gum is most often grown on a sugar solution substrate isolated from corn, soy, wheat, and in some cases, dairy. It is reliably gluten-free, and a study published in the journal *Allergy* noted that allergic reactions to gums based on their substrate are very rare.[30] However, if you are concerned about a highly sensitive food allergy, contact the manufacturer to confirm the substrate on which the xanthan gum was grown and avoid any trigger ingredients, or switch to using another option such as guar gum.

Starch vs. flour: keeping them straight

A source of potential confusion when shopping for blend ingredients is the use of the words *starch* and *flour.* For tapioca and arrowroot, they are interchangeable. For example, tapioca starch, tapioca flour, and the confusingly named tapioca starch flour are all the same thing. This is *not* true for potato and corn. Potato flour and corn flour are made from the whole, dehydrated food, while potato starch and cornstarch are made only from the isolated starch. They *cannot* be substituted for each another.

High-altitude adjustments

Any recipes that require adjustments for baking at high altitude have those instructions noted on the recipe itself.

How to store baked goods: getting the most out of gluten-free goodies

Gluten-free baked goods tend to go stale faster than their wheat-based counterparts. If you're not going to eat them fresh, within the first day or so, allow them to cool completely and then freeze. Skip the countertop and the refrigerator.

GF ARTISAN GLUTEN-FREE (GF) FLOUR BLEND

1 cup of Artisan GF Flour Blend weighs 125 g.

SINGLE BATCH

• MAKES ABOUT 3 CUPS •

1¼ cups (156 g) brown rice flour
¾ cup (88 g) sorghum flour
⅔ cup (90 g) cornstarch
¼ cup (37 g) potato starch
1 tablespoon plus 1 teaspoon (14 g) potato flour
1 teaspoon (3 g) xanthan gum

QUADRUPLE BATCH

• MAKES ABOUT 12 CUPS •

5 cups (625 g) brown rice flour
3 cups (350 g) sorghum flour
2⅔ cups (360 g) cornstarch
1 cup (148 g) potato starch
⅓ cup (56 g) potato flour
1 tablespoon plus 1 teaspoon (14 g) xanthan gum

Combine all ingredients and whisk well to mix thoroughly. Store in an airtight container for up to 3 months in the pantry or 6 months in the refrigerator.

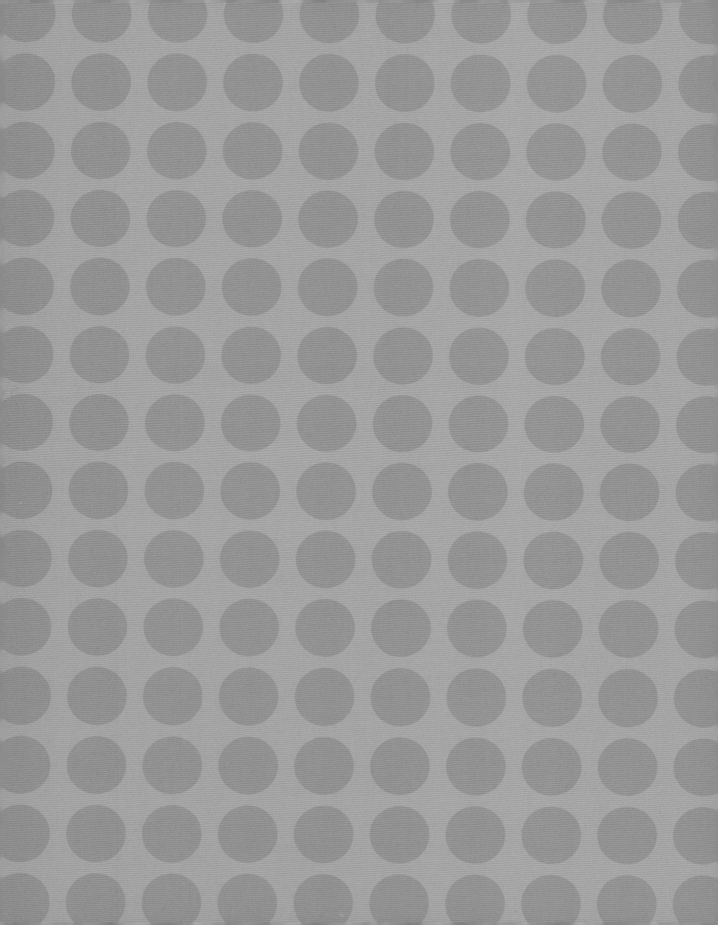

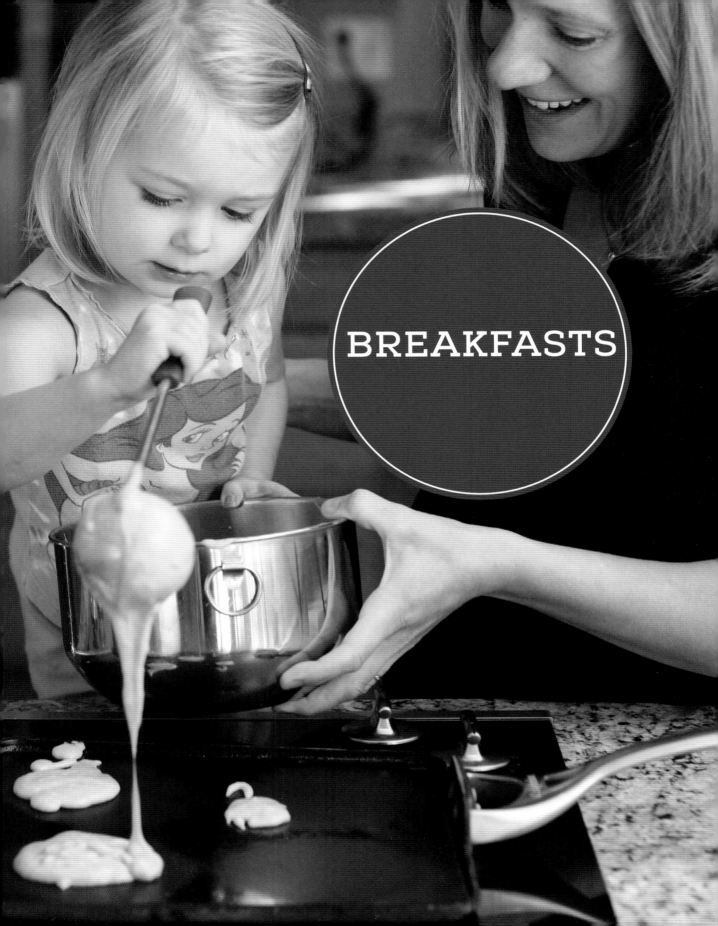

BREAKFASTS

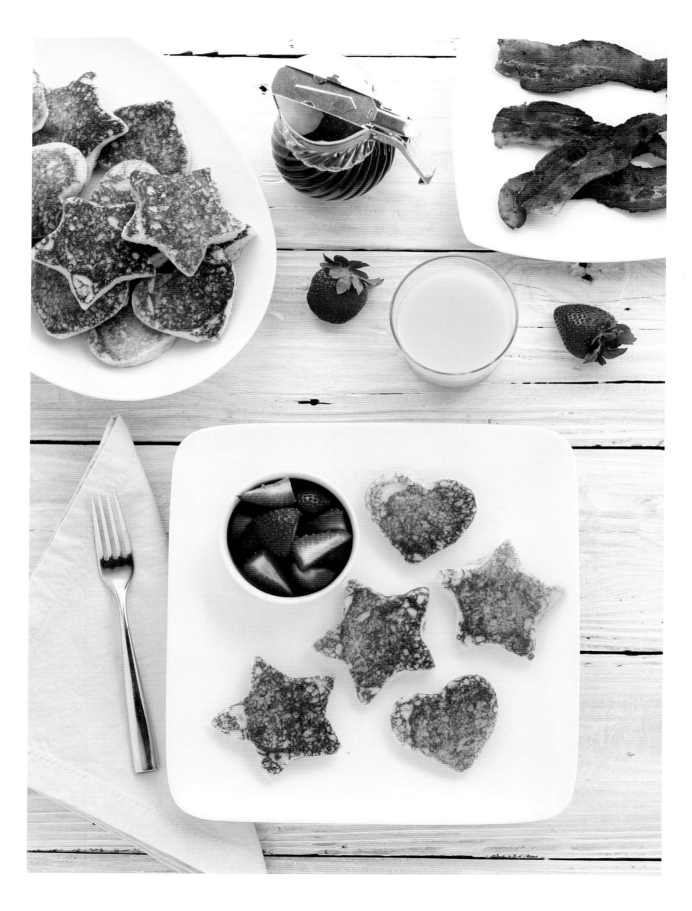

TRADITIONAL PANCAKES

• MAKES TWELVE 3-INCH (8 CM) PANCAKES •

These light and fluffy gluten-free pancakes are as good or better than their wheat-flour counter-parts. They're perfect for a weekend breakfast, breakfast-for-dinner, or any other time you love to whip up a batch. And to add some whimsy to this traditional dish, we make the pancakes using metal cookie cutters for fun shapes that will appeal to younger eaters. You could also use nonstick metal or silicone pancake molds (sold in many different shapes) made expressly for the purpose.

1 cup (125 g) Artisan GF Flour Blend (page 27)

2 teaspoons GF baking powder

¼ teaspoon salt

1 cup (240 ml) milk

1 egg

1 tablespoon pure maple syrup

1 teaspoon GF pure vanilla extract

2 tablespoons butter, melted

KIDS CAN . . .

* Collect ingredients from the pantry and refrigerator

* Measure ingredients

* Dump ingredients into mixing bowl

* Mix ingredients with a whisk, spoon, or fork

* Ladle batter onto the griddle

* Flip pancakes with a spatula

1. Whisk together the flour, baking powder, and salt in a bowl. Add the milk, egg, maple syrup, and vanilla and whisk. Add the melted butter and whisk just until combined.

2. Heat a griddle or skillet over medium-high heat. Grease the griddle and metal cookie cutters with butter or nonstick cooking spray.

3. Place the cookie cutters on the griddle and pour a small amount of batter into each, just enough to cover the bottom. Cook for about 30 seconds to set the edges of the pancakes. Carefully remove the cookie cutters (metal versions will get hot!) and continue to cook until bubbles form on the surface of each pancake. Flip and cook until the other side is golden brown. (Alternatively, omit the cookie cutters and simply pour the batter onto the griddle, using a 2-ounce/60 ml ladle or similar for traditional round pancakes.)

4. Repeat step 3 until the batter is used up. Re-grease the cookie cutters as needed to prevent sticking.

To make this recipe . . . .

EGG-FREE

* In a small bowl, combine 1 tablespoon ground flaxseeds and 3 tablespoons water. Allow the mixture to set for at least 2 minutes and use in place of the egg.

DAIRY/LACTOSE/CASEIN-FREE

* Substitute almond milk (or, for nut allergies, rice or hemp milk) for the cow's milk.
* Use 2 eggs instead of 1.
* Substitute melted coconut oil or melted vegan shortening for the butter.

CORN-FREE

* Use arrowroot flour to make a corn-free version of the Artisan GF Flour Blend (page 26).
* Check the ingredients of your baking powder, which often contains cornstarch.

VEGAN

* Use the dairy-free and egg-free substitutions.

SWEET POTATO PANCAKES

• MAKES SIXTEEN 3-INCH (8 CM) PANCAKES •

Whether you agree or not, a criticism of regular pancakes is that they're relatively empty nutrition-ally (notwithstanding that you can top them with all sorts of fresh fruit and other options). By add-ing sweet potato puree to pancake batter, you'll boost the pancakes' dietary fiber, potassium, and vitamin A, among other benefits. If making your own sweet potato puree, plan ahead and follow the roasting and pureeing directions below; otherwise, feel free to substitute store-bought puree.

1 cup (125 g) Artisan GF Flour Blend (page 27)

2 teaspoons GF baking powder

1 teaspoon ground cinnamon

¼ teaspoon salt

1 cup (240 ml) milk

½ cup (120 g) sweet potato puree (see below to make your own)

2 eggs

1 tablespoon pure maple syrup

2 tablespoons butter, melted

¼ cup (30 g) chopped pecans, optional

1. Whisk together the flour, baking powder, cinnamon, and salt in a bowl. Add the milk, sweet potato puree, eggs, and maple syrup and whisk until smooth. Add the melted butter and mix to combine. Mix in pecans if desired.

2. Heat a griddle or skillet over medium-high heat. Grease with butter or nonstick cooking spray.

3. Using a 2-ounce (60 ml) ladle or similar, pour the batter onto the hot griddle or skillet to make pancakes that are about 3 inches (8 cm) in diameter. Cook until bubbles have formed on the surface of the pancakes and the surface appears slightly dry. Flip and cook until the other side is golden brown.

4. Repeat step 3 until the batter is used up.

Make your own . . .

SWEET POTATO PUREE: Preheat the oven to 400°F (200°C). Using a fork, pierce the skin of a 5.5-ounce (156 g) sweet potato on all sides and place in a baking pan. Roast for 45 to 60 minutes, until you can easily stick a knife into the center and the flesh is very soft. When cool enough to handle, peel and puree in a food processor until smooth. Alternatively, use a potato masher or fork to get the sweet potato as smooth as possible. Makes about ½ cup (120 g) sweet potato puree. Alternatively, follow the same procedure with a 16-ounce (454 g) sweet potato to yield about 1½ cups (360 g) puree, and save the leftovers for another use.

KIDS CAN . . .

* Scrape the flesh from the potato skin and press the food processor buttons

* Collect ingredients from the pantry and refrigerator

* Measure ingredients

* Dump ingredients into mixing bowl

* Mix ingredients with a whisk, spoon, or fork

* Ladle batter onto the griddle

* Flip pancakes with a spatula

To make this recipe . . . .

EGG-FREE

● In a small bowl, combine 2 tablespoons ground flaxseeds and ¼ cup plus 2 tablespoons (90 ml) water. Allow the mixture to set for at least 2 minutes and use in place of the eggs.

DAIRY/LACTOSE/CASEIN-FREE

● Substitute almond milk (or, for nut allergies, rice or hemp milk) for the cow's milk.

● Substitute melted coconut oil or melted vegan shortening for the butter.

CORN-FREE

● Use arrowroot flour to make a corn-free version of the Artisan GF Flour Blend (page 26).

● Check the ingredients of your baking powder, which often contains cornstarch.

VEGAN

● Use the dairy-free and egg-free substitutions.

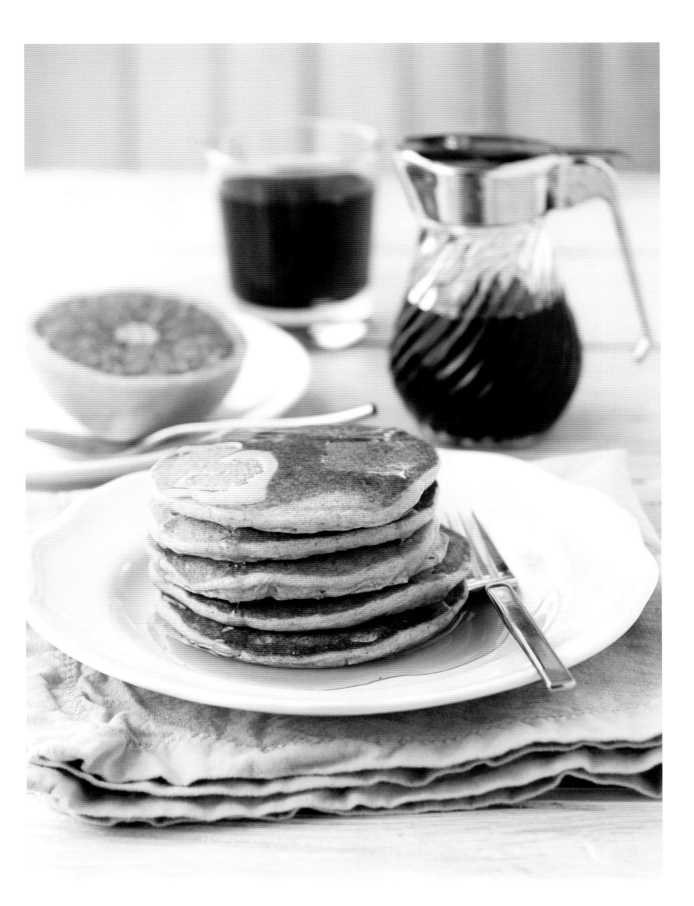

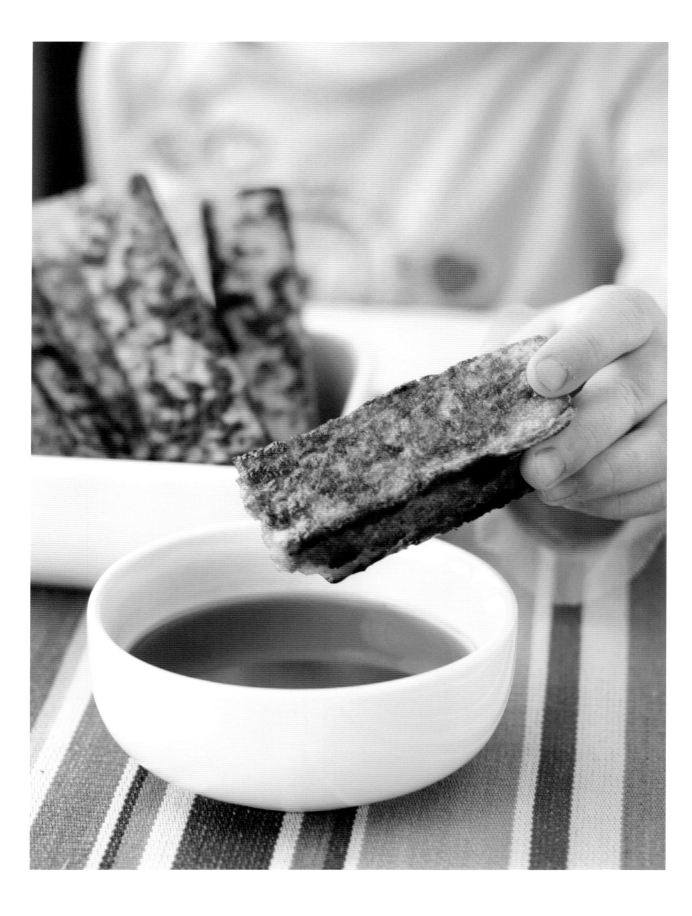

FRENCH TOAST STICKS

• MAKES 16 STICKS (4 SERVINGS) •

French toast sticks are classic kid food. Their "stick" format just invites children to pick them up with their hands, maybe dip an end in pure maple syrup, and take a bite. (Parents are welcome to do that, too!) Most store-bought gluten-free bread is sliced too thin and is the wrong texture to make really good French toast sticks. Using our Sandwich Bread recipe, however, will deliver excellent results!

Four 1-inch (2.5 cm) thick slices Sandwich Bread (page 80)

4 eggs

⅓ cup (80 ml) milk

1 teaspoon GF pure vanilla extract

½ teaspoon ground cinnamon

KIDS CAN . . .

* Collect ingredients from the pantry and refrigerator
* Cut the bread
* Measure ingredients
* Dump ingredients into mixing bowl
* Mix ingredients with a whisk, spoon, or fork
* Dip the bread pieces in egg mixture
* Set the dipped bread on the pan

1. Cut each slice of bread into 4 even strips to give you 16 sticks of bread. In a wide-bottomed bowl, whisk together the eggs, milk, vanilla, and cinnamon.

2. Heat a skillet or pancake pan over medium-high heat. Grease the pan with butter.

3. Dip the bread sticks into the egg mixture, coating all sides and allowing any excess to drip off. Place the sticks directly on the hot greased pan. Cook the sticks 1 to 2 minutes per side until all four sides are golden brown.

4. Repeat step 3 until all of the sticks are cooked.

NOTE: The refined-sugar-free, dairy/lactose/casein-free, and corn-free statuses of this recipe are partially dependent on the ingredients in your bread. Our Sandwich Bread (page 80) can be made any combination of the above.

To make this recipe . . . .

DAIRY/LACTOSE/CASEIN-FREE:

* Substitute almond milk (or, for nut allergies, rice or hemp milk) for the cow's milk.
* Use nonstick cooking spray, vegan shortening, or another nondairy option to grease the pan.

HOT CEREAL

• MAKES 3 CUPS •

Our girls are virtually addicted to gluten-free oatmeal. When we ask them what they'd like for break-fast, that's their answer four out of five times. But sometimes you need to branch out, and this hot ce-real really does the trick. It has the texture and quality of cream of wheat, but without the gluten. The millet makes the cereal high in magnesium, often deficient in those recovering from celiac disease.

¼ cup (48 g) brown rice

¼ cup (27 g) GF old-fashioned rolled oats

¼ cup (49 g) whole millet

4 cups (950 ml) water, apple juice, milk, or dairy-free milk

OPTIONAL TOPPINGS

Diced bananas, strawberries, peaches, and/or apples

Blueberries, raspberries, and/or raisins

Pure maple syrup, honey, or brown sugar

Ground cinnamon, toasted pecans, and/or flaxseeds

1. Use a spice grinder or high-power blender to grind the rice, oats, and millet to a powder. This can be done in batches if all of the ingredients do not fit.*

2. Place the cereal powder in a heavy saucepan and add the liquid. (Water will give you a base cereal, apple juice a slightly sweetened cereal, and milk a creamy cereal.) Bring to a simmer over high heat, whisking con-stantly. Turn the heat down to maintain a slow simmer and cook for 30 minutes, whisking frequently to pre-vent lumps from forming and the cereal from sticking to the bottom of the pan. Serve immediately with de-sired toppings.

*You can also grind larger batches of the grains ahead of time and store in an airtight container so that cereal is on hand and ready to cook. Instead of using ¼ cup each of brown rice, oats, and millet, use ¾ cup plus 2 tablespoons (125 g total) of the ground mixture.

VARIATIONS

If you want to boost the nutrition in this hot cereal, try either of these two options:

- **QUINOA HOT CEREAL:** To the existing blend of cereals, add ¼ cup (44 g) rinsed and dried quinoa, grinding it as the other cereals. Increase the liquid from 4 to 5 cups. The "super grain" quinoa adds a complete protein with the full complement of amino acids. The quinoa has a dominant flavor that transforms the hot cereal's profile.

- **AMARANTH HOT CEREAL:** To the existing blend of cereals, add ¼ cup (47 g) amaranth, grinding it as the other cereals. Increase the liquid from 4 to 5 cups. Amaranth is naturally high in the amino acid lysine, often lacking in grains such as rice and millet. By adding amaranth to the cereal, it will have the full complement of amino acids to make a complete protein.

KIDS CAN . . .

✳ Collect ingredients from the pantry and refrigerator

✳ Measure ingredients

✳ Press the "grind" button on the spice grinder or blender

✳ Dump ingredients into the saucepan

✳ Mix ingredients with a whisk

✳ Stir the pot occasionally while cooking

To make this recipe . . . .

TREE-NUT-FREE, REFINED-SUGAR-FREE, AND/OR VEGAN

- Avoid any toppings that do not meet these requirements.

DAIRY/LACTOSE/CASEIN-FREE

- Make sure to use water, apple juice, or non-dairy milk.

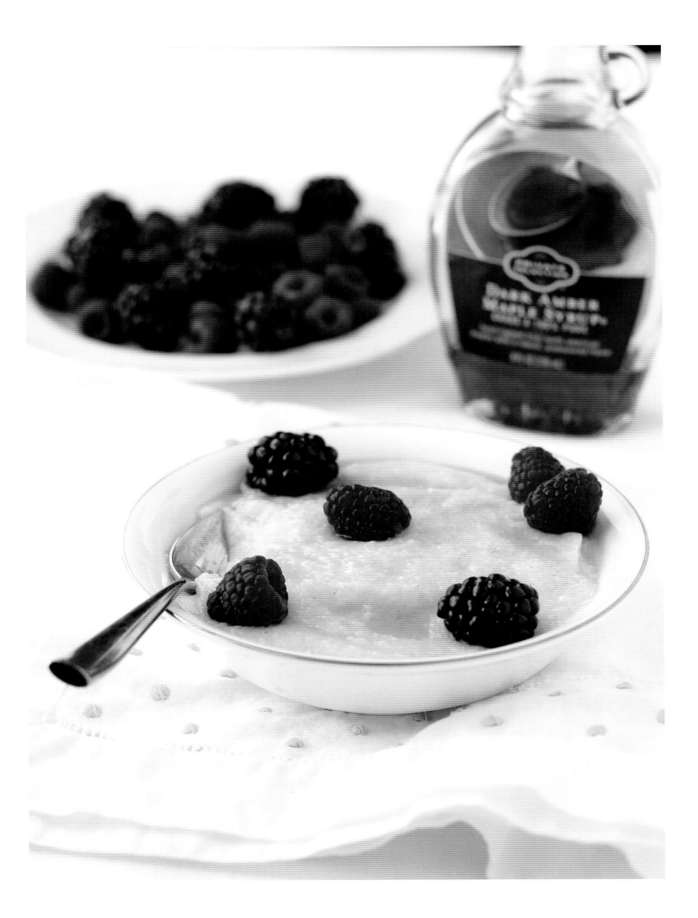

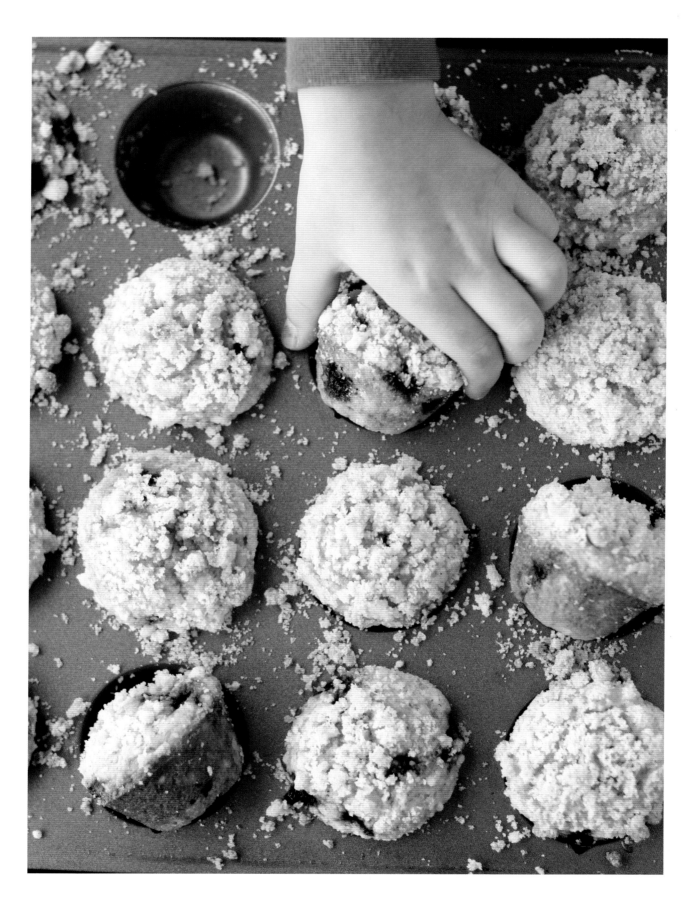

BLUEBERRY MINI MUFFINS

• MAKES 24 MINI MUFFINS •

These miniatures of the popular classic have a moist and tender crumb. You could easily substitute mini chocolate chips for the berries. When it's our turn to bring snack to our daughters' preschool classes, these mini muffins are always popular among the kids (and the teachers).

2 cups (250 g) Artisan GF Flour Blend (page 27)

1 teaspoon xanthan gum

1½ teaspoons GF baking powder

1 cup (216 g) sugar

½ cup (1 stick, 113 g) butter, melted

½ cup (120 ml) half-and-half

2 eggs

½ teaspoon GF pure vanilla extract

1 cup (125 g) frozen wild blueberries*

KIDS CAN . . .

* Collect ingredients from the pantry and refrigerator

* Grease the muffin tin and place liners if using

* Measure ingredients

* Dump ingredients into the mixing bowl

* Mix ingredients with a spoon

* Scoop the batter into prepared muffin tin

1. Preheat the oven to 400°F (200°C). Grease the cups of a 24-cup mini muffin tin with butter or nonstick cooking spray. Place paper liners in the greased cups if desired.

2. In a medium bowl, mix together the flour, xanthan gum, baking powder, and sugar. Add the melted butter and stir to form a crumbled mixture. Set aside ½ cup of the mixture for the topping.

3. In a separate bowl, mix together the half-and-half, eggs, and vanilla. Add to the crumbled mixture, stirring just until moist to make a batter. Fold the blueberries into the batter.

4. Scoop the batter into the prepared muffin cups. A cookie scoop works very well to transfer the batter. Sprinkle the tops of the muffins with the reserved crumble mixture.

5. Bake for 12 to 15 minutes, until the muffins spring back when lightly pressed and a toothpick comes out clean. The muffins should be slightly golden brown on top. Let the muffins cool in the tins for 5 minutes, then remove and serve.

*The fresh blueberries typically available in season are too big for these mini muffins. Instead, we prefer smaller wild blueberries, which are usually only available in the freezer section.

To **make this recipe** . . . .

EGG-FREE

● In a small bowl, combine 2 tablespoons ground flaxseeds and 1/4 cup plus 2 tablespoons (90 ml) water. Allow the mixture to set for at least 2 minutes and use in place of the eggs.

DAIRY/LACTOSE/CASEIN-FREE

● Add ¼ teaspoon salt to the flour mixture.

● Substitute melted coconut oil for the butter.

● Substitute cashew cream (see page 44 to make your own) for the half-and-half.

CORN-FREE

● Use arrowroot flour to make a corn-free version of the Artisan GF Flour Blend (page 26).

● Check the ingredients of your baking powder, which often contains cornstarch.

VEGAN

● Use the dairy-free and egg-free substitutions.

BANANA MINI MUFFINS

• MAKES 24 MINI MUFFINS •

If your family is like ours, you go through phases with bananas. One week they're eaten in no time; another they sit on the counter for days, threatening to go over the hill at any moment. Before they do, let this recipe come to your bananas' rescue. Our preference is to use bananas that are crossing over toward over-ripe status, with plenty of brown spots, which makes them nice and sweet and soft.

3 medium-size, ripe bananas

1 egg

½ cup (170 g) honey

¼ cup (59 g) applesauce

1 teaspoon GF pure vanilla extract

1½ cups (188 g) Artisan GF Flour Blend (page 27)

1 teaspoon xanthan gum

1½ teaspoons GF baking powder

¼ teaspoon baking soda

¼ teaspoon salt

1 teaspoon ground cinnamon

1. Preheat the oven to 350°F (175°C). Grease the cups of a 24-cup mini muffin tin with butter or nonstick cooking spray. Place paper liners in the greased muffin cups, if desired.

2. Mash the bananas in a large bowl until mostly smooth with a few large lumps. (A stand mixer is ideal for this job, using the paddle attachment.) Mix in the egg, honey, applesauce, and vanilla.

3. In a separate bowl, combine the flour, xanthan gum, baking powder, baking soda, salt, and cinnamon, whisking to mix well. Add the dry ingredients to the banana mixture and mix at low speed just until combined, 5 to 10 seconds. Scrape down the sides of the bowl and mix at high speed for about 5 seconds, until the batter is thoroughly mixed.

4. Scoop the batter into the prepared muffin cups. A cookie scoop works very well to transfer the batter. Bake for 15 to 18 minutes, until the muffins spring back when lightly touched and a toothpick comes out clean. The muffins should be slightly golden brown on top. Let the muffins cool in the tin for 5 minutes, then remove and serve.

KIDS CAN . . .

* Collect ingredients from the pantry and refrigerator

* Grease the muffin tin and place liners if using

* Measure ingredients

* Dump ingredients into the mixing bowl

* Whisk dry ingredients

* Scoop the batter into prepared muffin tin

To **make this recipe** . . . .

EGG-FREE AND VEGAN

* In a small bowl, combine 1 tablespoon ground flaxseeds and 3 tablespoons water. Allow the mixture to set for at least 2 minutes and use in place of the egg.

CORN-FREE

* Use arrowroot flour to make a corn-free version of the Artisan GF Flour Blend (page 26).
* Check the ingredients of your baking powder, which often contains cornstarch.

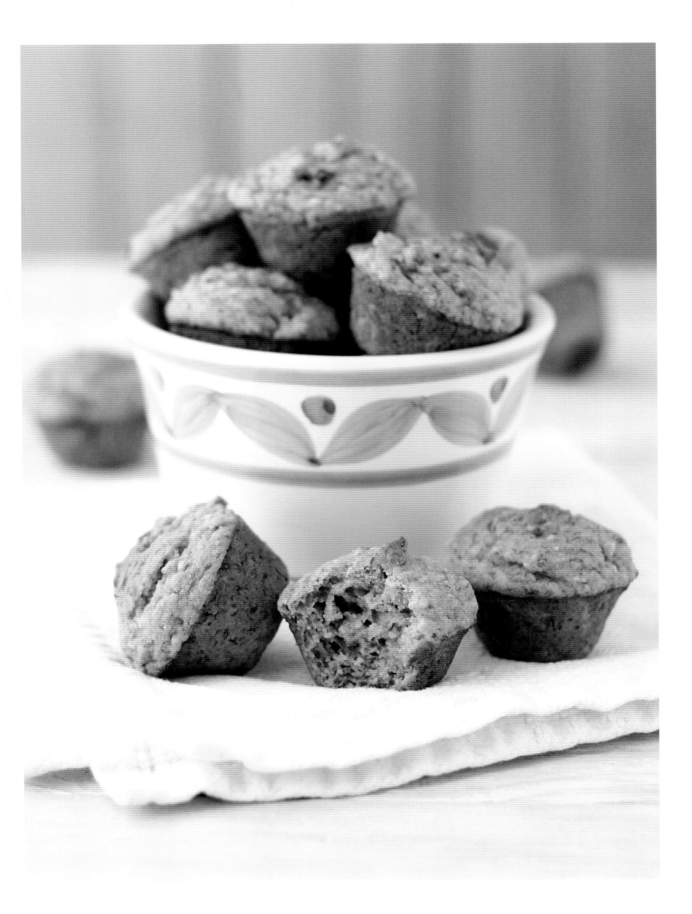

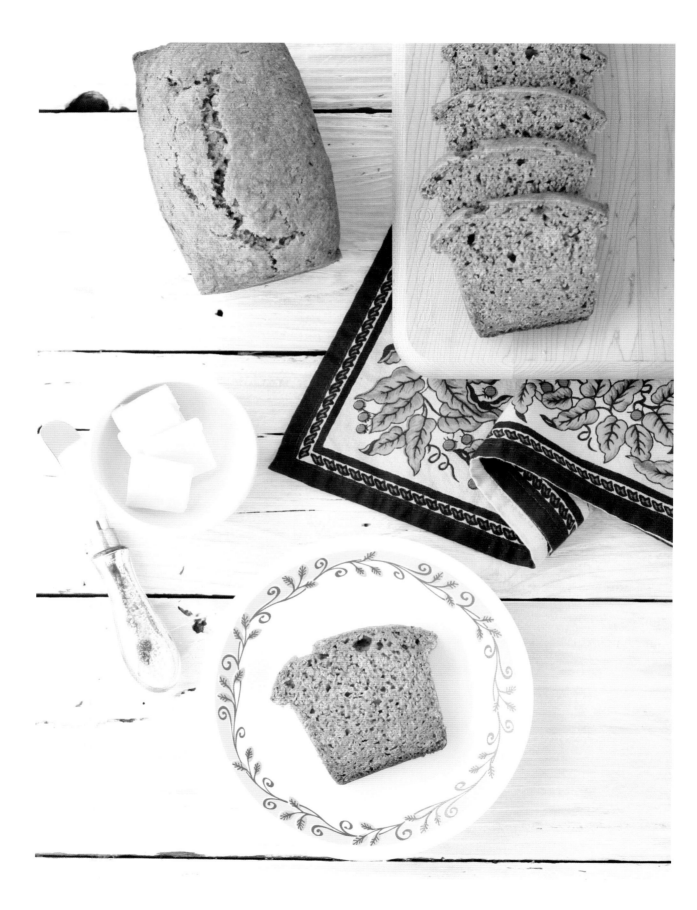

ZUCCHINI BREAD

• MAKES 3 MINI LOAVES OR 1 LARGE LOAF •

This zucchini bread—packed with fresh zucchini and a hint of spice—has a super moist and tender crumb. If your kids are at all like ours, they'll eat it as quickly as you can make it! The recipe's taken on added significance for us in recent years, ever since our younger daughter, Charlotte, learned to walk among the rows of our community garden plot back in New York's Hudson Valley, which yielded an amazing bounty of zucchini.

3 cups (375 g) Artisan GF Flour Blend (page 27)

1 teaspoon xanthan gum

1 teaspoon GF baking powder

½ teaspoon baking soda

2 teaspoons ground cinnamon

¼ teaspoon ground nutmeg

½ teaspoon salt

2 cups (240 g) finely grated zucchini
   (1 large zucchini)

½ cup (115 g) packed brown sugar

½ cup (170 g) honey

½ cup (118 g) applesauce

½ cup (120 ml) coconut oil

3 eggs

1. Preheat the oven to 350°F (175°C). Grease three 3 x 5-inch (8 x 13 cm) mini loaf pans* or one 5 x 9-inch (13 x 23 cm) loaf pan with oil or nonstick cooking spray.

2. Combine the flour, xanthan gum, baking powder, baking soda, cinnamon, nutmeg, and salt in a bowl and whisk to combine. In a separate bowl, combine the zucchini, brown sugar, honey, applesauce, coconut oil, and eggs, whisking to combine. Add the flour mixture to the zucchini mixture, stirring until the flour is just incorporated.

3. Divide the batter among the prepared mini loaf pans (or scrape into the large loaf pan), smoothing the tops with a wet spatula. Bake the mini loaves for 45 minutes (or the large loaf for 70 to 80 minutes), until a toothpick inserted in the center of each loaf comes out clean.

4. Allow to cool in the pan(s) for 10 minutes, then flip out of the pan(s) onto a wire rack to cool completely.

*If your mini loaf pans are smaller than 3 x 5 inches (8 x 13 cm), use four pans.

KIDS CAN . . .

✳ Collect ingredients from the pantry and refrigerator

✳ Measure ingredients

✳ Dump ingredients into the mixing bowl

✳ Mix the ingredients with a whisk

✳ Divide the batter among the pans and smooth the tops

To make this recipe . . . .

EGG-FREE
- In a small bowl, combine 3 tablespoons ground flaxseeds and 1/2 cup plus 1 tablespoon water (135 ml). Allow the mixture to set for at least 2 minutes and use in place of the eggs.

CORN-FREE
- Use arrowroot flour to make a corn-free version of the Artisan GF Flour Blend (page 26).
- Check the ingredients of your baking powder, which often contains cornstarch.

VEGAN
- Follow the egg-free instructions and substitute agave nectar for the honey.

SCONES

Whether you're British or not, you can appreciate these rich gluten-free scones, made with either chocolate chips or blueberries. Perhaps due to the English heritage on Kelli's side of the family, our girls do love a scone with a spot of tea—decaf black, with milk and sugar. Such refined little ladies! Store any leftover scones in an airtight container for up to 3 days on the counter or freeze for up to 1 month.

1¾ cups (219 g) Artisan GF Flour Blend (page 27)

1 tablespoon GF baking powder

1 teaspoon xanthan gum

¼ teaspoon salt

¼ cup (54 g) sugar

6 tablespoons (¾ stick, 84 g) butter

½ cup (90 g) mini chocolate chips (or frozen wild blueberries, 63 g)

½ cup (120 ml) half-and-half

1 egg

½ teaspoon GF pure vanilla extract

1. Preheat the oven to 375°F (190°C).

2. Mix the flour, baking powder, xanthan gum, salt, and sugar in a bowl. Cut the butter into the flour mixture with a pastry blender or your hands until the mixture resembles pea-size crumbles. Add the chocolate chips (or blueberries) to the flour mixture and toss to combine.

3. In a separate bowl, whisk together the half-and-half, egg, and vanilla. Add to the flour mixture and stir until a dough forms. The dough will be slightly sticky; you can add a few tablespoons of additional flour to make the dough easier to work with if desired.

4. Form the dough into a log about 12 inches (30 cm) long. Press on the log to flatten and spread to 3 inches (8 cm) wide. Press along the length to square the sides. Cut the dough crosswise in half, and then divide each half into three 2 x 3-inch (5 x 8 cm) rectangles. Cut each rectangle diagonally to form triangles.

5. Place the scones on an ungreased baking sheet. Bake for 12 minutes, until light golden brown. Allow the scones to cool on the baking sheet before serving.

Make your own . . .

CASHEW CREAM: Soak 1 cup (148 g) raw cashew pieces in water overnight. Drain and rinse the nuts. Put in your blender with 2 cups (475 ml) cold water. Blend about 4 minutes (unless you have a professional-grade machine, which will blend faster), until completely smooth. Makes 3 cups (710 ml).

KIDS CAN . . .

* Collect ingredients from the pantry and refrigerator

* Measure ingredients

* Dump ingredients into the mixing bowl

* Mix the butter into the flour mixture with hands

* Whisk together the wet ingredients

* Shape and cut scones

* Place scones on baking sheet

To make this recipe . . . .

EGG-FREE

● In a small bowl, combine 1 tablespoon ground flaxseeds and 3 tablespoons water. Allow the mixture to set for at least 2 minutes and use in place of the egg.

DAIRY/LACTOSE/CASEIN-FREE

● Substitute vegan shortening for the butter.

● Confirm that your chocolate chips (if using) do not contain dairy.

● Substitute ¾ cup cashew cream (see above to make your own) for the ½ cup half-and-half.

CORN-FREE

● Use flour to make a corn-free version of the Artisan GF Flour Blend (page 26).

● Check the ingredients of your baking powder, which often contains cornstarch.

REFINED-SUGAR-FREE

● Substitute coconut sugar for the granulated sugar.

VEGAN

● Use the dairy-free and egg-free substitutions.

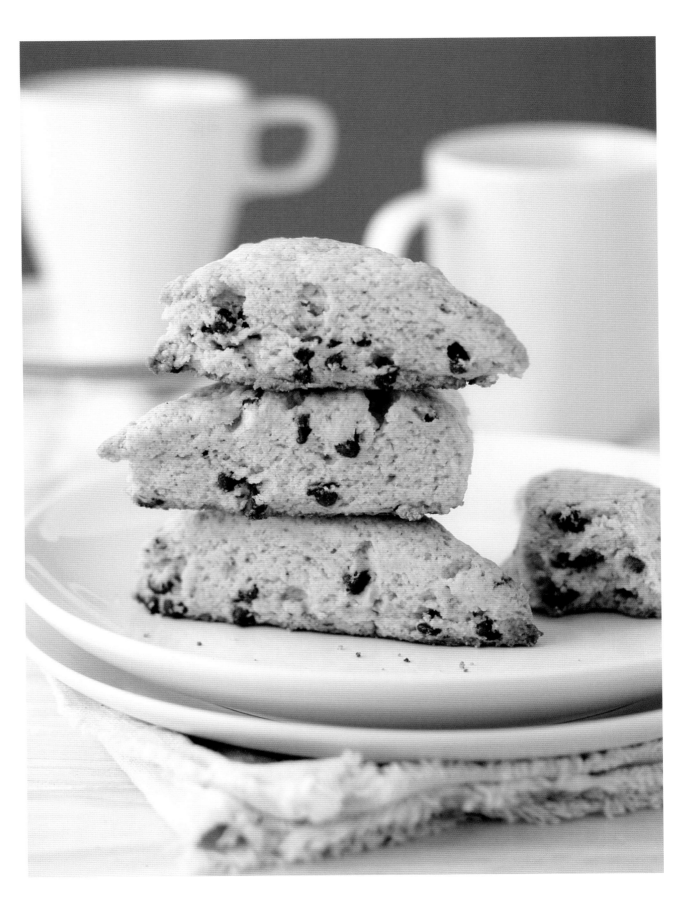

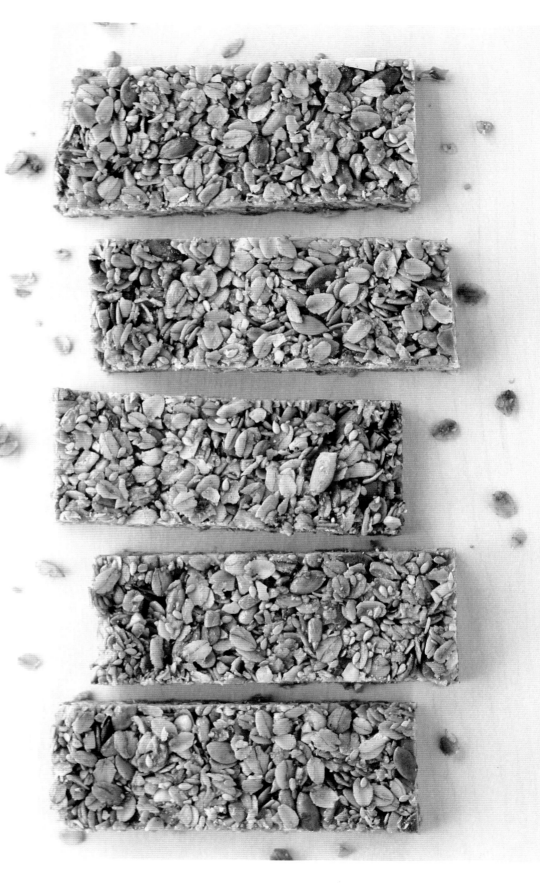

CINNAMON GRANOLA BARS

• MAKES 12 BARS •

These nutritious bars travel well and are great either as part of breakfast or as an easy, portable snack to enjoy throughout the day. Feel free to experiment with different nuts and seeds as well as dried fruit to change up the flavors. Or make it into Crumbled Granola (see below) that's great with yogurt or milk, or spooned over Cinnamon Apples (page 64) to make a faux apple crisp.

¾ cup (96 g) blanched almonds

3 cups (324 g) GF old-fashioned rolled oats

½ cup (75 g) raw pepitas (hulled pumpkin seeds)

½ cup (72 g) raw sunflower seeds

¼ cup (38 g) golden flaxseeds

2 teaspoons ground cinnamon

¼ teaspoon ground nutmeg

¼ teaspoon ground ginger

1 teaspoon salt

¾ cup (250 g) agave nectar

½ cup (120 ml) olive oil

1 teaspoon GF pure vanilla extract

½ cup (80 g) chopped dried fruit, optional

½ cup (90 g) mini chocolate chips, optional

KIDS CAN . . .

* Collect ingredients from the pantry and refrigerator

* Crush almonds

* Measure ingredients

* Dump ingredients into the mixing bowl

* Stir the mixture with a spoon

* Spread the mixture in the baking pan

1. Preheat the oven to 350°F (175°C). Line a 13 x 9-inch (33 x 23 cm) baking pan with parchment paper.

2. Place the blanched almonds in a zip-top bag and use a mallet, rolling pin, or bottom of a heavy pan to crush into small pieces.

3. Combine the crushed almonds, oats, pepitas, sunflower seeds, flaxseeds, cinnamon, nutmeg, ginger, and salt in a large bowl and stir to combine. Pour on the agave nectar, olive oil, and vanilla extract and mix until evenly incorporated. Spread the mixture in the prepared baking pan. Bake for 15 minutes.

4. Turn the oven down to 300°F (150°C). Stir the granola in the pan and add the dried fruit and/or chocolate chips, if desired. Press the mixture firmly into the pan using a spatula. Bake an additional 25 minutes, until the top is golden.

5. Allow to cool completely, at least 2 hours. Cut into rectangles with a serrated knife. Store in an airtight container, separated by parchment paper, for up to 1 week at room temperature or up to 2 weeks in the refrigerator.

VARIATION

CRUMBLED GRANOLA: Preheat the oven to 325°F (165°C) and line a 13 x 18-inch (33 x 46 cm) rimmed baking sheet with parchment paper. Spread the granola mixture (without the dried fruit or chocolate chips) on the prepared baking sheet and bake for 15 minutes. Stir thoroughly and bake for an additional 15 minutes, until golden brown. Allow to cool completely. Crumble to form a loose granola, adding in any dried fruit and/or chocolate chips as desired. Makes 5 to 6 cups. Store in an airtight container in the refrigerator for up to 2 weeks.

To make this recipe . . . .

TREE-NUT-FREE
* Omit the almonds and optionally substitute additional seeds.

DAIRY/LACTOSE/CASEIN-FREE
* Confirm that your mini chocolate chips (if using) do not contain dairy.

HASH BROWN PATTIES

• MAKES 4 PATTIES •

Like our French Toast Sticks (page 35), Chicken Fingers (page 128), and other recipes, these hash brown patties serve up two things kids love best: straightforward flavors and finger food. They're delicious on their own or lightly dipped in ketchup. And unlike hash brown patties from the freezer section of your supermarket and fast food franchises, these contain only three familiar ingredients.

1 pound (454 g) russet potatoes (about 3 small potatoes)

2 to 4 tablespoons olive oil

Salt

KIDS CAN . . .

∗ Collect ingredients from the pantry and refrigerator

∗ Peel potatoes

∗ Shred potatoes

∗ Squeeze water from raw potatoes

1. Peel the raw potatoes and shred with a large-holed grater. Fill a medium bowl with cold water, submerge the shredded potatoes, and soak for 2 minutes. Drain the potatoes and place in a clean kitchen towel, mesh bag (such as a nut bag, usually used for squeezing nut milk out of nut pulp), or paper towels. Squeeze out as much water as possible. This will give you crispy, rather than mushy, potatoes.

2. Heat a large sauté pan over medium-high heat. Add 2 tablespoons olive oil to the heated pan. Grease the insides of four 3¾-inch (10 cm) rings (English muffin rings or tuna fish cans with both ends cut off) with olive oil or nonstick cooking spray and place in the pan.

3. Divide the potatoes between the four rings, about ½ cup shredded potato per ring, and season lightly with salt. Place a drinking glass with a large flat bottom on top of each. The base of the glass should be just slightly smaller than the ring so that it sits on and compresses the potatoes. Cook for 7 to 10 minutes, carefully rotating every few minutes to promote even browning.

4. Remove the glasses and rings and flip the patties. Clean off any potato sticking to the rings and replace the rings around each patty to help them hold their shape. Add 1 to 2 tablespoons olive oil to the pan if needed (too little oil will cause the patties to burn instead of brown and crisp). Season this side lightly with salt and replace the drinking glasses. Cook for an additional 7 to 10 minutes, rotating again for even browning, until deep golden brown and crispy at the edges. Remove the glasses, rings, and patties from the pan. Serve warm.

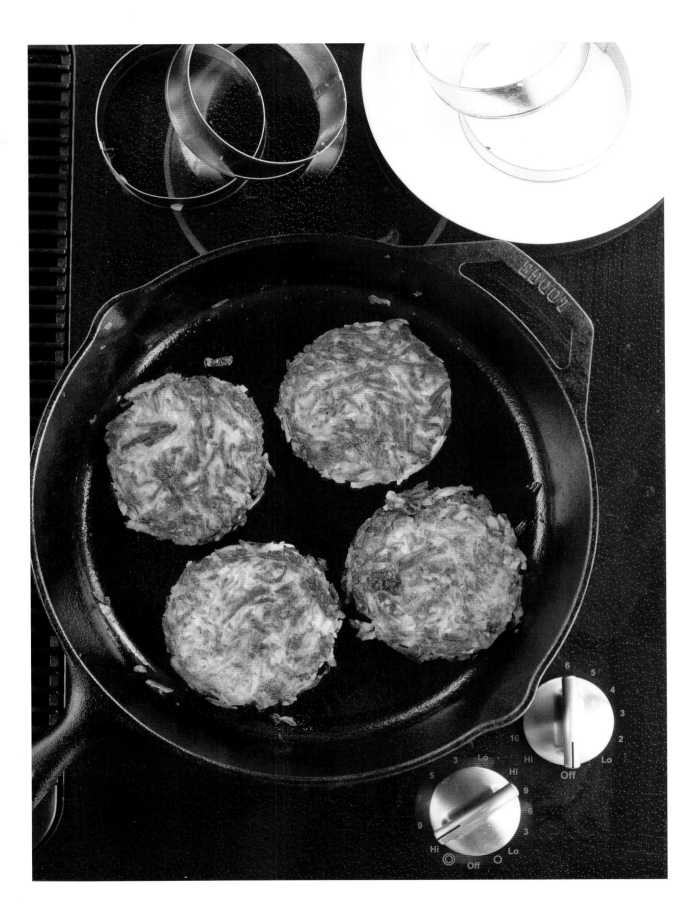

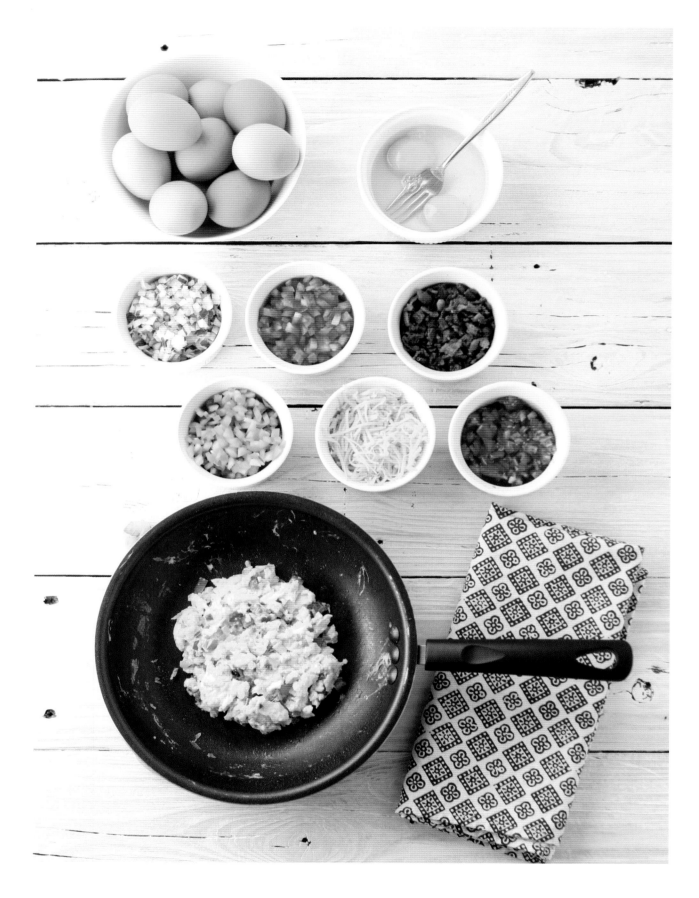

SCRAMBLED OMELETS

• MAKES ENOUGH OMELETS FOR THE FAMILY •

Scrambled omelets are a great way to use up leftovers and pack in a few extra veggies! We like to put out a number of options in small bowls for everyone in the family to pick their own add-ins to personalize their omelet.

2 eggs per omelet

1 tablespoon milk per omelet

Salt and pepper

SELECTION OF ADD-INS

Diced peppers, onions, mushrooms, and/or spinach

Small broccoli florets

Diced tomato, avocado, scallions, sun-dried tomatoes, olives, and/or ham

Bacon

Shredded feta, cheddar, or Swiss cheese

Smoky Tomato Salsa (page 107)

GF hot sauce

1. In a small bowl, whisk together 2 eggs, 1 tablespoon milk, and salt and pepper to taste.

2. Select and prepare any of your add-in ingredients: Heat a sauté pan over medium-high heat. Sauté any vegetables that require it first, using 1 to 2 teaspoons of olive oil. Then steam or wilt any vegetables, using a few tablespoons of water and cooking until the water is evaporated. Finally, if using bacon, cook until crispy, then drain the excess fat from the pan. Have any fresh ingredients that don't require preparation ready to go as well.

3. To make an omelet: Grease the pan with olive oil or nonstick cooking spray and heat over medium-high heat. Add the egg mixture to the hot pan along with add-ins of choice. Use a spatula to scramble by agitating the egg and mixing the toppings together. Cook until all parts of the egg are dry, about 3 minutes.

4. Repeat the process for each person's own personalized omelet. Or scale up the recipe (2x, 3x, etc.) and make one large omelet to portion off and share.

KIDS CAN . . .

﹡ Collect ingredients from the pantry and refrigerator

﹡ Prep toppings, for example, slice mushrooms, dice avocado, shred cheese

﹡ Measure ingredients

﹡ Dump ingredients into mixing bowl

﹡ Mix ingredients with a whisk, spoon, or fork

To **make this recipe** . . . .

DAIRY/LACTOSE/CASEIN-FREE
- Substitute water for the cow's milk.
- Only use nondairy toppings.

VEGETARIAN
- Only use vegetarian options (e.g., no bacon or ham!).

PERSONAL QUICHES

• MAKES 12 INDIVIDUAL QUICHES •

Perfect for little hands to hold and bite, these personal quiches are fun to make and eat. They also store well in the refrigerator and reheat easily in the microwave or toaster oven, making them a great make-ahead breakfast option.

CRUST

1⅓ cups (167 g) Artisan GF Flour Blend (page 27)

¼ teaspoon salt

¼ cup (½ stick, 56 g) butter

1 egg

¼ cup (60 ml) cold water

1 teaspoon apple cider vinegar

FILLING

3 eggs

½ cup (120 ml) half-and-half

¼ cup (60 ml) milk

Salt and pepper

¾ to 1 cup (80 to 130 g) diced vegetables, cooked meat, and/or cheese

KIDS CAN ...

* Collect ingredients from the pantry and refrigerator

* Measure ingredients

* Dump ingredients into the mixing bowl

* Mix butter/shortening into flour mixture with hands

* Whisk together the wet ingredients

* Press the dough into the muffin tins

* Divide the filling among the muffin tins

* Pour the egg mixture into the prepared cups

1. To make the crust: In a large bowl, mix together the flour and salt. Cut the butter into the flour using a pastry blender or your hands until it resembles fine crumbs. Mix together the egg, water, and vinegar. Make a well in the flour mixture and pour the wet ingredients inside. Mix together with a spoon and then by hand until a dough forms. Wrap the dough in plastic wrap and refrigerate for 30 minutes.

2. Preheat the oven to 350°F (175°C). Grease the cups of a 12-cup muffin tin with butter or nonstick cooking spray.

3. Divide the dough into 12 equal portions and place one in each muffin cup. Use the plastic wrap the dough was wrapped in to press each piece of dough to cover the bottom and three-fourths up the sides of each cup. The plastic wrap helps prevent the dough from sticking to your fingers.

4. To make the filling: Combine the eggs, half-and-half, milk, salt, and pepper in a bowl, whisking to combine.

5. Place 1 to 1½ tablespoons vegetables, cooked meat, and/or cheese in each cup. Pour the egg mixture into each cup, filling it to just below the edge of the dough. Bake the quiches for 40 minutes, until the egg is slightly puffed and golden brown.

6. Allow the quiches to cool for 10 minutes, then use a knife to carefully cut around each crust (to make sure it isn't stuck to the tin) and pop the quiches out of the tin.

To make this recipe...

DAIRY/LACTOSE/CASEIN-FREE
* For the crust, substitute vegan shortening for the butter.
* For the filling, substitute almond milk (or, for nut allergies, rice or hemp milk) for the half-and-half and milk.

CORN-FREE
* Use arrowroot flour to make a corn-free version of the Artisan GF Flour Blend (page 26).

VEGETARIAN
* Use only vegetarian fillings.

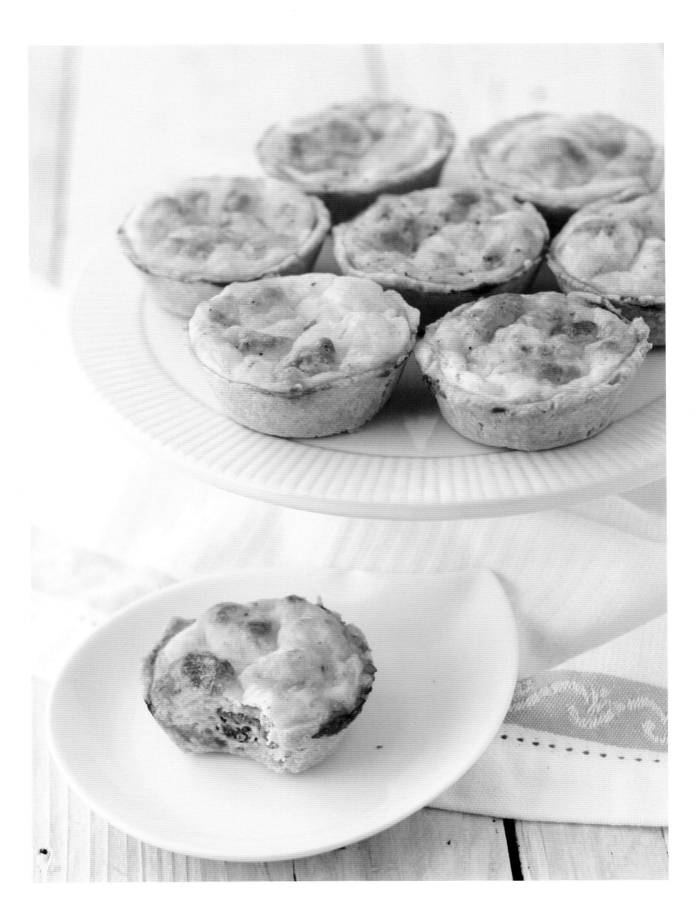

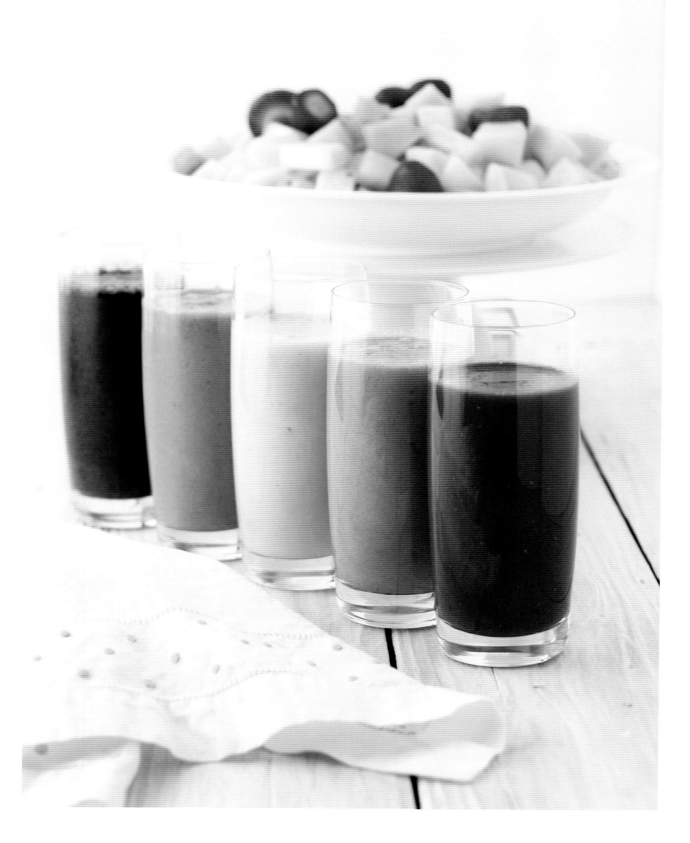

RAINBOW OF SMOOTHIES

• EACH SMOOTHIE RECIPE MAKES 2½ TO 3 CUPS •

Smoothies are a wonderful way to pack tons of nutrition—including fresh fruits and vegetables, and the fiber that comes with them—into a delicious beverage kids love. Plus, their bright crayon-like colors make them even more fun. We buy fruits and vegetables when they're fresh and in season (and on sale)—bananas, berries, spinach, peaches, melons—then cut them up and freeze for use throughout the year.*

PINK SMOOTHIE

1 ripe banana, cut into chunks

1 small beet, peeled and cut into pieces

10 strawberries, hulled

½ cup (120 ml) cashew or almond milk

½ cup (65 g) crushed ice

ORANGE SMOOTHIE

10 baby carrots

1 cup (160 g) chopped cantaloupe

1 ripe banana, cut into chunks

½ cup (120 ml) orange juice

½ cup (65 g) crushed ice

YELLOW SMOOTHIE

1 cup (178 g) chopped pineapple

1 golden apple or peach, cored or pitted and cut into pieces

1 ripe banana, cut into chunks

½ cup (120 ml) milk

½ cup (65 g) crushed ice

GREEN SMOOTHIE

2 cups (90 g) packed baby spinach

1 banana, cut into chunks

1 cup (180 g) chopped honeydew

½ cup (120 ml) orange juice

½ cup (65 g) crushed ice

PURPLE SMOOTHIE

1 ripe banana, cut into chunks

1 cup (125 g) frozen blueberries

1 cup (45 g) packed baby spinach

½ cup (120 ml) almond milk

½ cup (65 g) ice

Blend all ingredients until smooth.

*Whether we're talking strawberries, cantaloupe, or another fruit, to freeze, remove the leaves, stems, seeds, rind, etc. Cut into pieces, spread in a single layer on a baking sheet, and pop in the freezer until completely frozen. Then transfer to another container for more compact, longer-term storage in the freezer.

KIDS CAN . . .

* Collect ingredients from refrigerator

* Place ingredients in the measuring cup

* Peel and slice fruit (such as banana)

* Count items (such as strawberries or baby carrots)

* Place ingredients in blender

* Press buttons on blender

To make this recipe . . . .

TREE-NUT-FREE

• If the smoothie calls for cashew or almond milk, substitute soy or cow's milk (which introduces dairy).

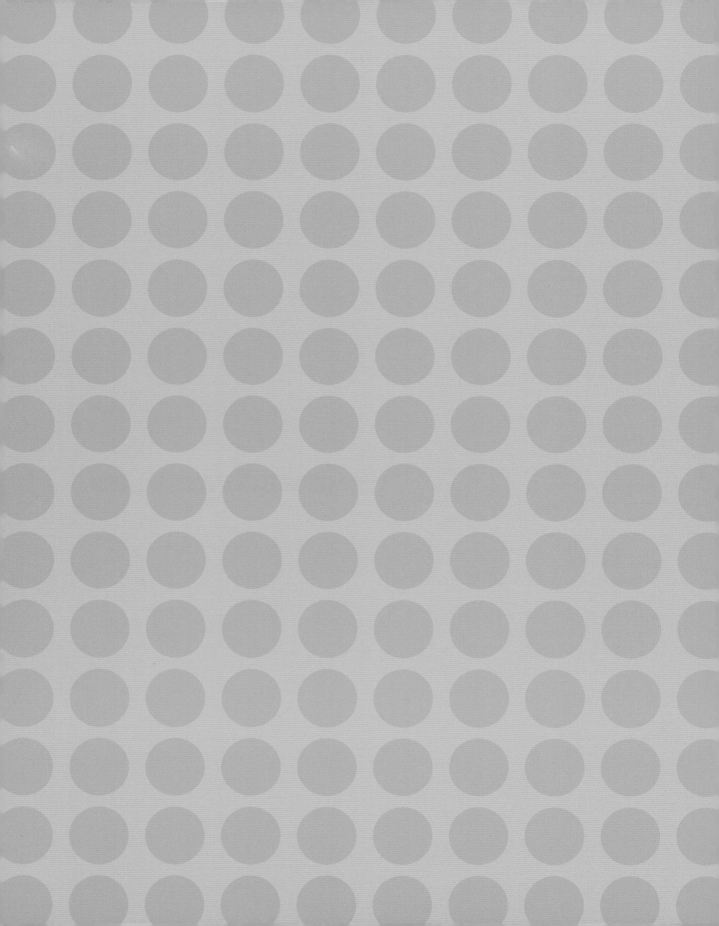

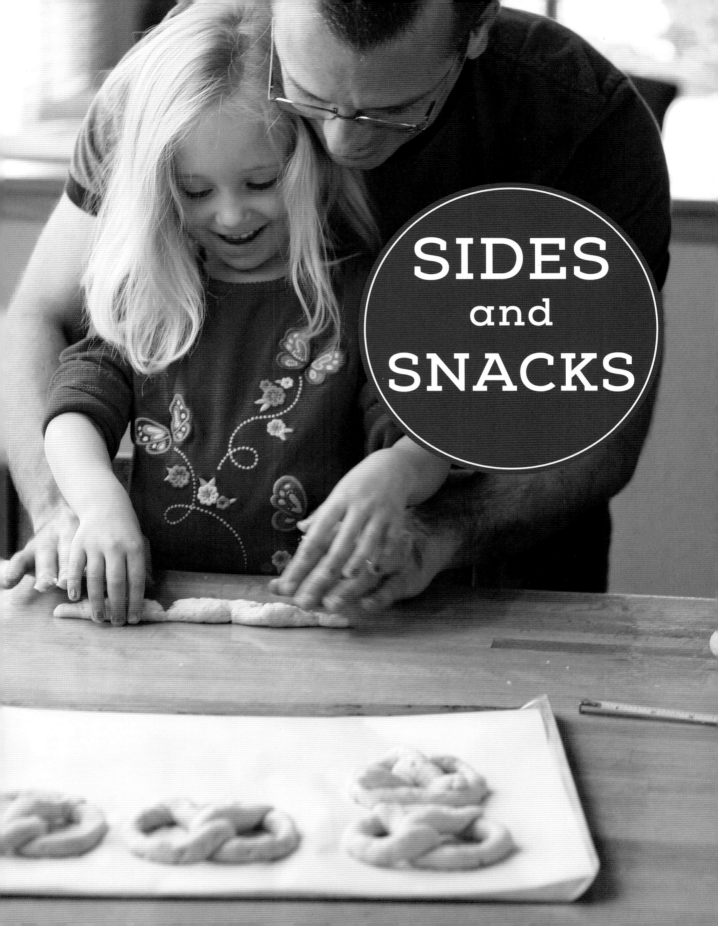

SIDES
and
SNACKS

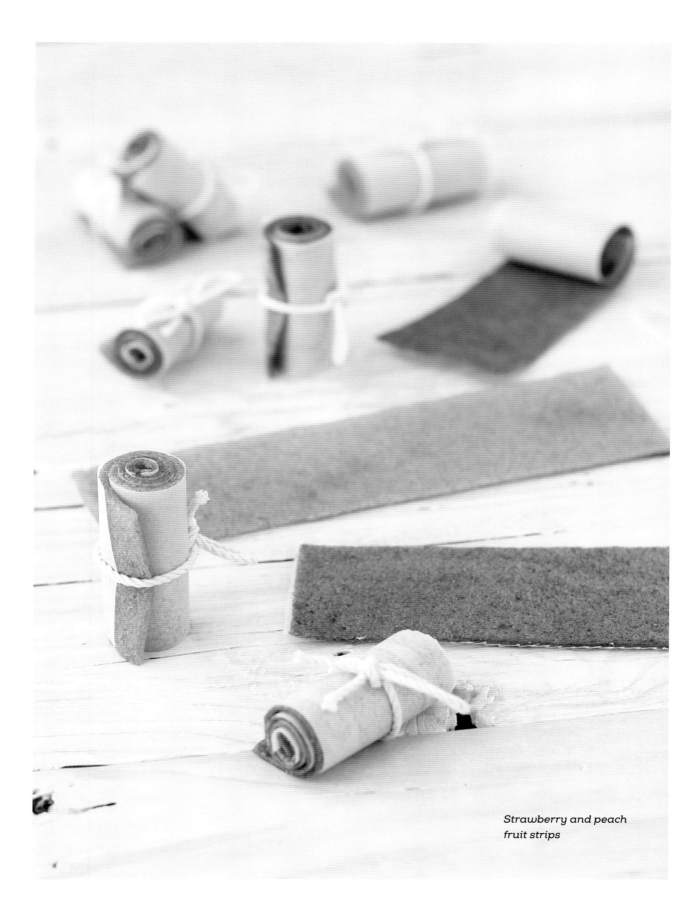

Strawberry and peach fruit strips

FRUIT STRIPS

• MAKES FIVE 2 X 8-INCH (5 X 20 CM) STRIPS •

With just three ingredients, these homemade fruit strips are as simple as can be. They are chewy and fun, just like the store-bought varieties, but without all of the additional, hard-to-pronounce ingredients. This recipe is easily doubled.

2 cups (about 300 g) cut-up fruit (e.g., about 3 peaches, 2 mangos, or ⅔ quart strawberries)

Juice of ½ lemon (about 2 tablespoons)

Agave nectar, honey, or sugar, optional

KIDS CAN . . .

* Collect ingredients from the pantry and refrigerator

* Cut up fruit with an age-appropriate knife

* Measure ingredients

* Use citrus reamer to juice lemon over strainer to catch seeds

* Dump ingredients into food processor

* Press the food processor buttons

* Roll up the cut strips

1. Preheat the oven to 170°F (75°C). Line a 13 x 9-inch (33 x 23 cm) baking pan with parchment paper cut to fit just to the edges, or with a silicone baking mat.

2. Puree the fruit and lemon juice in the food processor until smooth. Taste to see how sweet the puree is and, if desired, add a sweetener, bearing in mind that the flavor intensifies as the fruit dries. Using an offset spatula or similar utensil, spread the pureed fruit into a thin layer to cover the entire pan.

3. Bake the fruit puree for 5 to 6 hours, rotating every hour or so to dry evenly. When the fruit is nearly completely set, and just slightly sticky, remove from the oven and allow to cool.

4. When the fruit is cool, remove from the pan and, if desired, transfer to a clean sheet of parchment paper that is the same size as the fruit. Using sharp kitchen scissors or a knife, trim the edges to make them completely straight. Cut the fruit and parchment paper together into 2-inch (5 cm) strips, then cut each strip into desired length. Roll up the strips, including the parchment, and store in an airtight container for up to 1 month.

NOTES: If you happen to over-bake the fruit (it gets dry and cracks when you try to roll it, instead of leathery and pliable), simply spritz it with water or brush lightly with a wet pastry brush to partially rehydrate. Let sit for a few minutes before handling.

To double the recipe, increase the fruit from 2 to 4 cups and use an 11 x 16-inch pan with a lip.

To make this recipe . . . .

REFINED-SUGAR-FREE
* If you decide to sweeten the fruit puree, use honey or agave nectar and not sugar.

VEGAN
* If you decide to sweeten the fruit puree, use agave nectar or sugar and not honey.

FRUIT KABOBS WITH YOGURT FONDUE

• MAKES 1½ CUPS (355 ML) FONDUE •

This creamy and slightly sweet fondue is reminiscent of cheesecake filling. Fruit kabobs empower kids to make their own fruit combinations, and it's fun to dip kabobs in the fondue. Or enjoy the yogurt fondue with Crumbled Granola (page 47).

4 ounces (113 g) cream cheese, room temperature

1 cup (240 g) Greek yogurt

3 tablespoons honey

Juice of ½ lemon (about 2 tablespoons)

½ teaspoon GF pure vanilla extract

½ cantaloupe

½ honeydew melon

½ pineapple

1 quart (600 g) strawberries

1. In a bowl, beat the cream cheese with a handheld mixer until smooth. Add the yogurt, honey, lemon juice, and vanilla and beat until completely incorporated. Transfer to a serving bowl.

2. Cut the cantaloupe, honeydew, and pineapple into 1-inch (2.5 cm) pieces. Wash the strawberries and cut off the green tops.

3. Slide the fruit onto wooden skewers (you can do this ahead of time, or each family member can make their own skewers in the moment as you eat). Serve the skewers with the yogurt fondue.

KIDS CAN ...

* Collect ingredients from the pantry and refrigerator

* Measure ingredients

* Dump ingredients into mixing bowl

* Juice the lemon using a citrus reamer over strainer to catch the seeds

* Help an adult hold the mixer to combine ingredients

* Cut the fruit with an age-appropriate knife

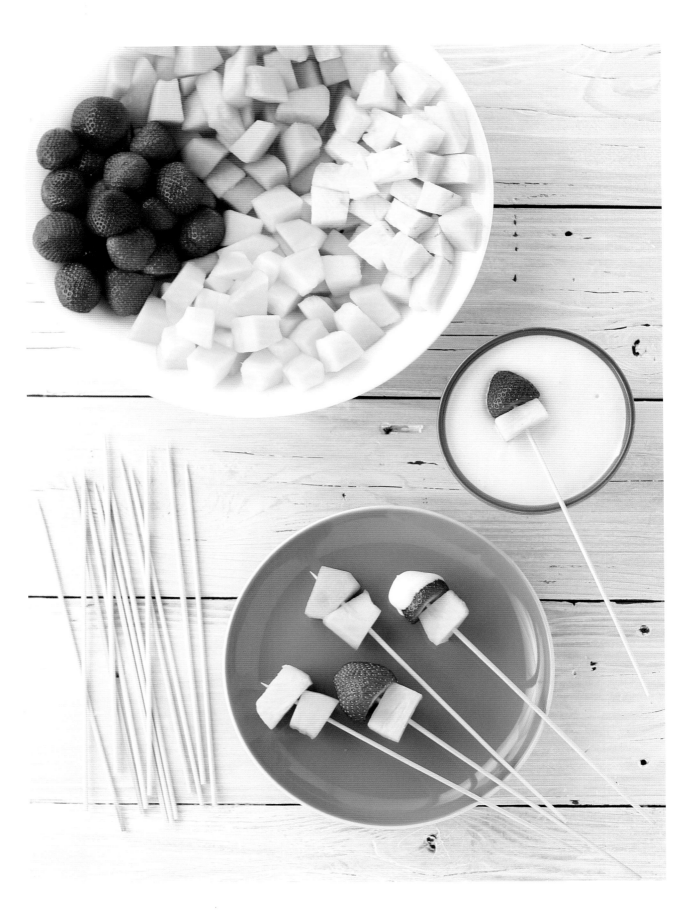

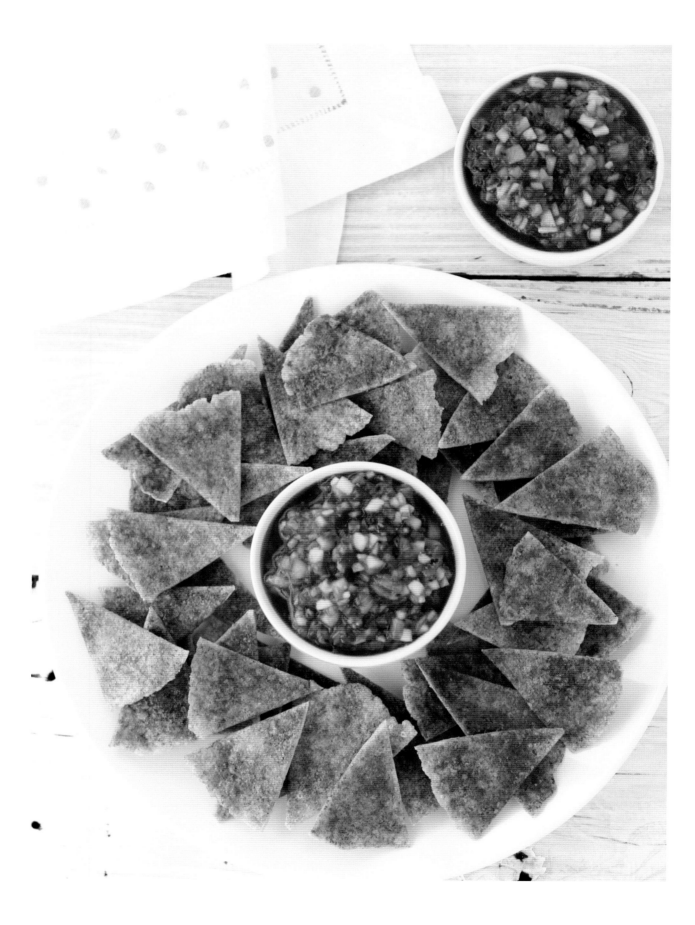

FRUIT SALSA WITH CINNAMON CHIPS

• MAKES 2 CUPS (475 ML) SALSA AND ABOUT 100 CHIPS •

An alternative to traditional chips and salsa, this fruit and cinnamon chip duo can be served as a snack or even as an appetizer.

FRUIT SALSA

8 strawberries, diced small

1 kiwi, diced small

½ Granny Smith apple, diced small

5 mint leaves, minced

Juice of ½ lemon (about 2 tablespoons)

½ to 1 tablespoon sugar, agave nectar, or honey, optional (based on the fruit's sweetness)

CINNAMON CHIPS

2 tablespoons sugar

2 teaspoons ground cinnamon

Tortilla Sandwich Wraps (page 112; twelve 5-inch/13 cm tortillas)

3 tablespoons butter, melted

1. To make the fruit salsa: Combine all of the salsa ingredients in a bowl, cover, and refrigerate until serving.

2. Preheat the oven to 375°F (190°C).

3. To make the cinnamon chips: Mix the sugar and cinnamon together in a small bowl. Brush each tortilla with melted butter and sprinkle with the cinnamon sugar. Cut each tortilla into 8 wedges. In batches, place the wedges in a single layer on an ungreased baking sheet and bake for 7 to 9 minutes, until the tortilla wedges are crispy and just starting to curl.

KIDS CAN . . .

* Collect ingredients from the pantry and refrigerator
* Dice the strawberries and kiwis
* Dump ingredients into mixing bowl
* Juice the lemon using a citrus reamer over strainer to catch the seeds
* Mix fruit salsa ingredients with a spoon
* Measure and mix cinnamon and sugar
* Brush tortillas with butter/coconut oil
* Sprinkle cinnamon sugar on tortillas

To make this recipe . . . .

DAIRY/LACTOSE/CASEIN-FREE
- Substitute melted coconut oil for the butter.

CORN-FREE
- Follow instructions to make the corn-free version of the Tortilla Sandwich Wraps (page 112).

REFINED-SUGAR-FREE
- Use agave nectar or honey, not sugar, in the fruit salsa.
- Substitute coconut sugar for the granulated sugar in the cinnamon chips.

VEGAN
- Substitute melted coconut oil for the butter.
- Use agave nectar or sugar for the sweetener.

CINNAMON APPLES

• MAKES 5 SERVINGS •

These cinnamon apples taste almost like apple pie filling and are so versatile: they're great on their own as a naturally sweet snack, topped with Crumbled Granola (page 47) to make a faux apple crisp, or enjoyed over pancakes or ice cream.

5 Granny Smith apples, peeled, cored, and sliced into 12 slices each

3 tablespoons butter

½ cup (170 g) honey or agave nectar

1½ teaspoons ground cinnamon

1 teaspoon ground nutmeg

1. Heat a sauté pan over medium-high heat. Add the apples, butter, and honey and cook for 2 minutes.

2. Add the cinnamon and nutmeg, cover, and simmer for 5 minutes.

3. Uncover, stir, and cook an additional 3 to 5 minutes, until the apples are soft and the liquid is syrupy.

KIDS CAN . . .

* Collect ingredients from the pantry and refrigerator

* Measure ingredients

* Dump ingredients in the pan

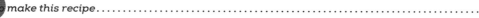

To make this recipe . . . .

DAIRY/LACTOSE/CASEIN-FREE

• Substitute melted coconut oil for the butter.

VEGAN

• Substitute melted coconut oil for the butter.

• Use agave nectar, not honey, for the sweetener.

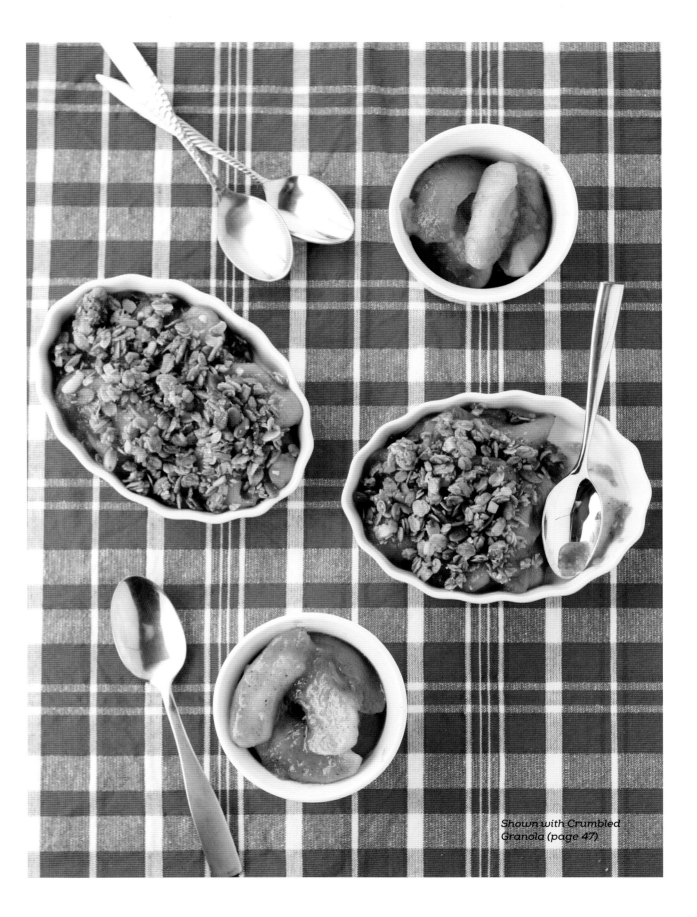

Shown with Crumbled Granola (page 47)

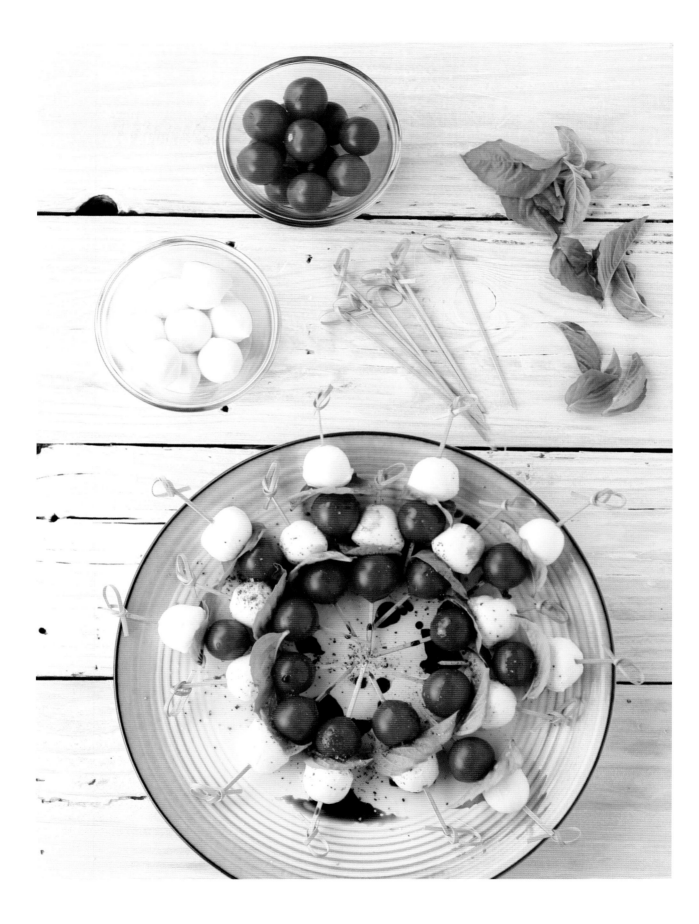

CAPRESE POPS

With a combination of fresh basil, tomato, and mozzarella, this salad-on-a-stick is a little piece of summer. Even young palates can enjoy the colorful, classic salad.

1 pint (about 25) cherry-size fresh mozzarella balls (sometimes called bocconcini)

Leaves from 1 bunch fresh basil (about 25 leaves)

1 pint (about 25) cherry tomatoes

1 to 2 tablespoons balsamic vinegar

1 to 2 tablespoons olive oil

Salt and pepper

1. Skewer one piece of mozzarella on a small bamboo skewer, then one basil leaf, and finally one cherry tomato. Repeat with the remaining ingredients to make 25 skewers and place them on a platter.

2. Drizzle the skewers with vinegar and olive oil and season with salt and pepper.

KIDS CAN . . .

* Collect ingredients from the pantry and refrigerator

* Skewer ingredients

* Drizzle vinegar and olive oil

HUMMUS

Hummus is a versatile, guilt-free dip that can be flavored many different ways. It is a great source of protein, fiber, and healthy fat. When our children were very young they stopped dipping vegetables and crackers in hummus, opting instead for a bowl and spoon, and they continue to eat it that way to this day!

One 15-ounce (425 g) can no-salt-added garbanzo beans, drained, liquid reserved; or 1½ cups (300 g) cooked beans, cooking liquid reserved

¼ cup (60 ml) olive oil

Juice of ½ lemon (about 2 tablespoons)

2 tablespoons tahini

1 small garlic clove, peeled

Salt

1. Combine the garbanzo beans, ¼ cup (60 ml) reserved liquid from the bean can or bean cooking liquid, olive oil, lemon juice, tahini, and garlic in a food processor.

2. Blend until very smooth, for about 2 minutes. Season with salt to taste.

VARIATIONS

SUN-DRIED TOMATO HUMMUS: Add ¼ cup (20 g) oil-packed sun-dried tomatoes and increase the reserved liquid and olive oil from ¼ cup (4 tablespoons) to 5 tablespoons each. If using dry sun-dried tomatoes, rehydrate them first by soaking in hot water for 30 to 60 minutes.

CILANTRO HUMMUS: Substitute lime juice for the lemon juice and add ½ teaspoon ground cumin and ½ cup (23 g) packed fresh cilantro.

KIDS CAN . . .

* Collect ingredients from the pantry and refrigerator

* Measure ingredients

* Put ingredients in food processor

* Juice the lemon/lime using a citrus reamer over strainer to catch the seeds

* Press the food processor buttons

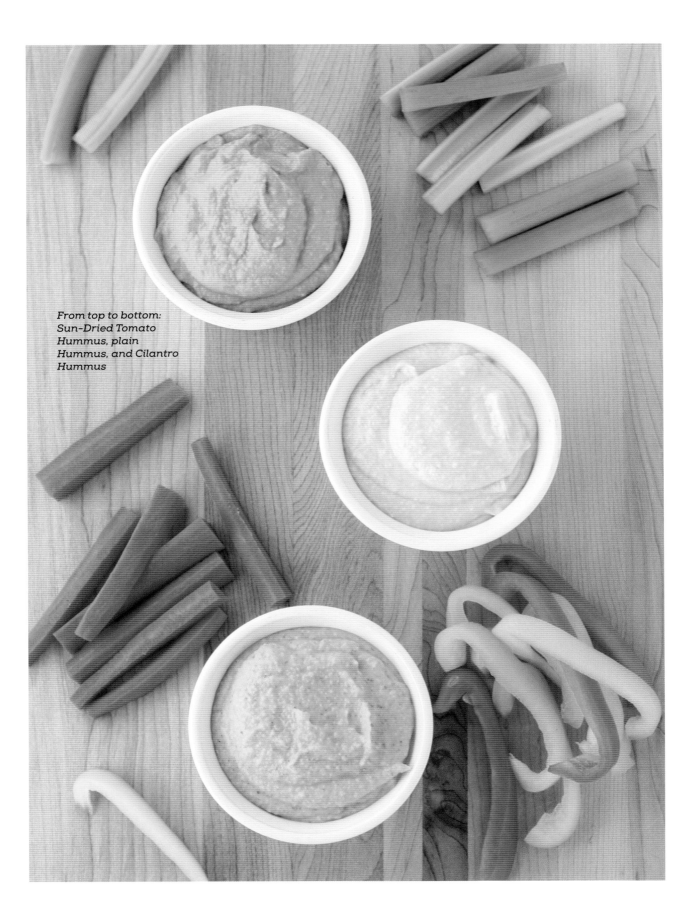

From top to bottom: Sun-Dried Tomato Hummus, plain Hummus, and Cilantro Hummus

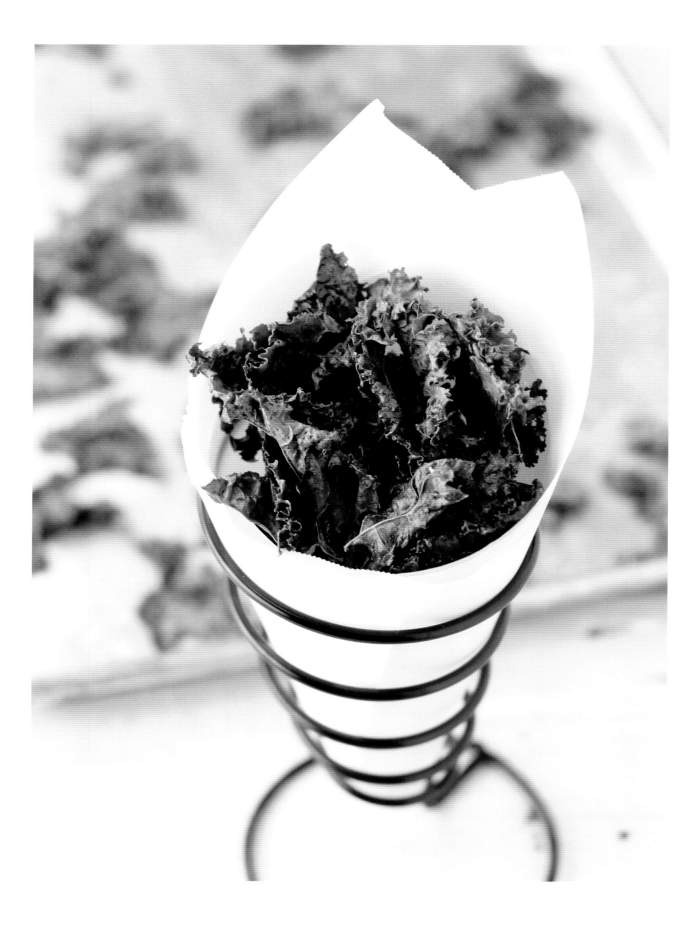

KALE CHIPS

• MAKES 4 TO 6 SERVINGS •

Before we had children, we'd never have believed that young kids would eat the "mature" flavors of kale chips. Boy, were we wrong! If we don't quickly snag some of this super vegetable snack for ourselves, we won't get any! These chips are 100 percent kid-friendly and guilt-free.

1 bunch (200 to 250 g) kale

1 to 2 tablespoons olive oil, depending on the size of your kale bunch

Sea salt

OPTIONAL ADDITIONAL SEASONINGS

Curry powder

Cinnamon and sugar

Chili powder and ground cumin

KIDS CAN ...

* Collect ingredients from the pantry and refrigerator

* Remove stems from kale and tear into pieces

* Rinse and dry kale

* Transfer kale to baking sheet

* Drizzle olive oil and seasoning

* Mix with hands

1. Preheat the oven to 275°F (135°C).

2. Remove the stems of the kale and tear the leaves into bite-size pieces. Rinse the kale in a colander and spread out on a kitchen towel. Roll up the towel to thoroughly dry the kale.

3. Transfer the kale to a baking sheet and drizzle with the olive oil. Toss with your hands to evenly coat with the oil. Arrange the kale in a single layer, dividing between 2 baking sheets if needed, and season lightly with salt and additional seasonings, if desired.

4. Bake for 25 minutes, until crisp. (Bake in batches if dividing between sheets.) They're best enjoyed the day of but can be stored in an airtight container for a day or two, though kale chips are notorious for turning from crisp to soggy when you do.

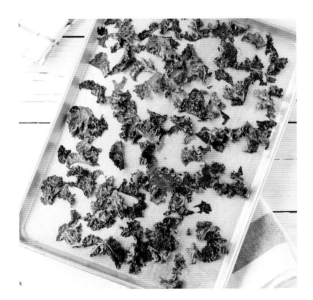

BRUSSELS BITES

• MAKES 4 TO 6 SERVINGS •

Brussels sprouts have long been maligned as the most-hated vegetable of children everywhere . . . until now. Gone are the days of mushy, boiled, flavorless Brussels sprouts! These are oven-roasted with a touch of garlic powder to create bite-size morsels that are almost like savory candy, and they will disappear like candy, too!

1½ pounds (680 g) whole Brussels sprouts

¼ cup (60ml) olive oil

¾ teaspoon garlic powder

½ teaspoon salt

½ teaspoon pepper

KIDS CAN . . .

* Collect ingredients from the pantry and refrigerator

* Transfer cut Brussels sprouts from cutting board to roasting pan

* Measure ingredients

* Drizzle the olive oil

* Sprinkle the seasonings

* Toss the ingredients together

1. Preheat the oven to 375°F (190°C).

2. Wash the Brussels sprouts and trim the ends. Cut the sprouts into halves or quarters, depending upon their size. Place in a large roasting pan in a single layer and drizzle with the olive oil. Add the garlic powder, salt, and pepper and toss to evenly coat.

3. Roast for 20 minutes. Remove from the oven and toss. Test for doneness and seasoning, adding more olive oil (if they are too dry) and additional seasoning to taste as necessary. Roast an additional 5 to 10 minutes, depending on the brownness and desired degree of doneness. We like a few dark leaves, golden-brown faces (cut sides), and an overall texture that rides the line between soft and al dente.

NOTE: You can also follow this same process for roasting cauliflower, after cutting the head into small florets.

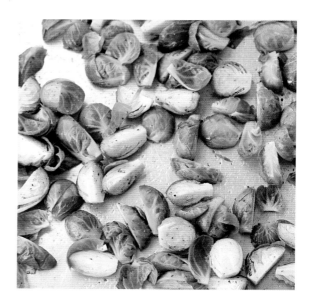

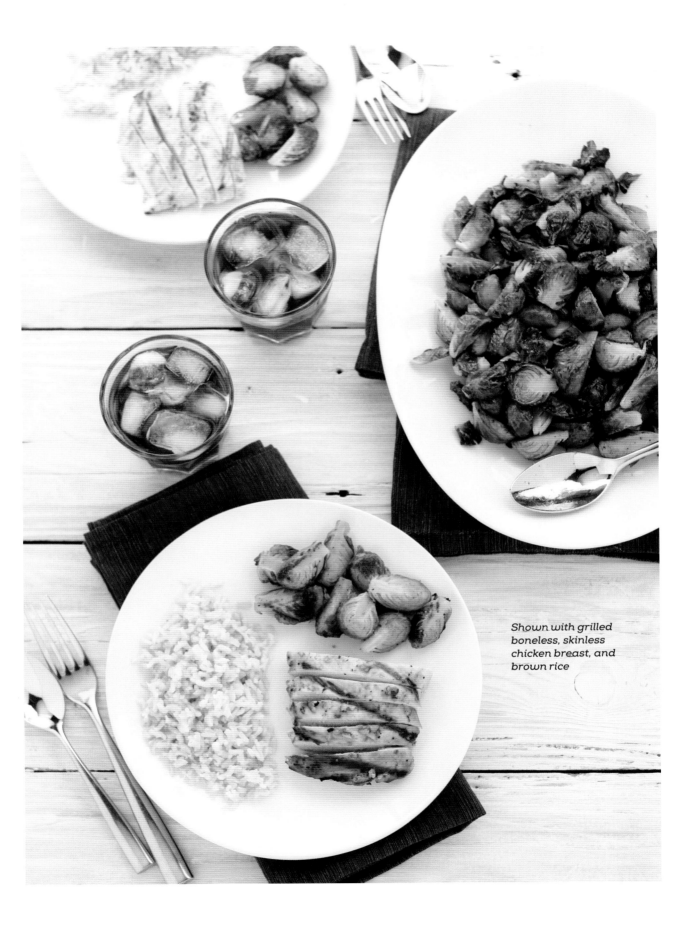

Shown with grilled boneless, skinless chicken breast, and brown rice

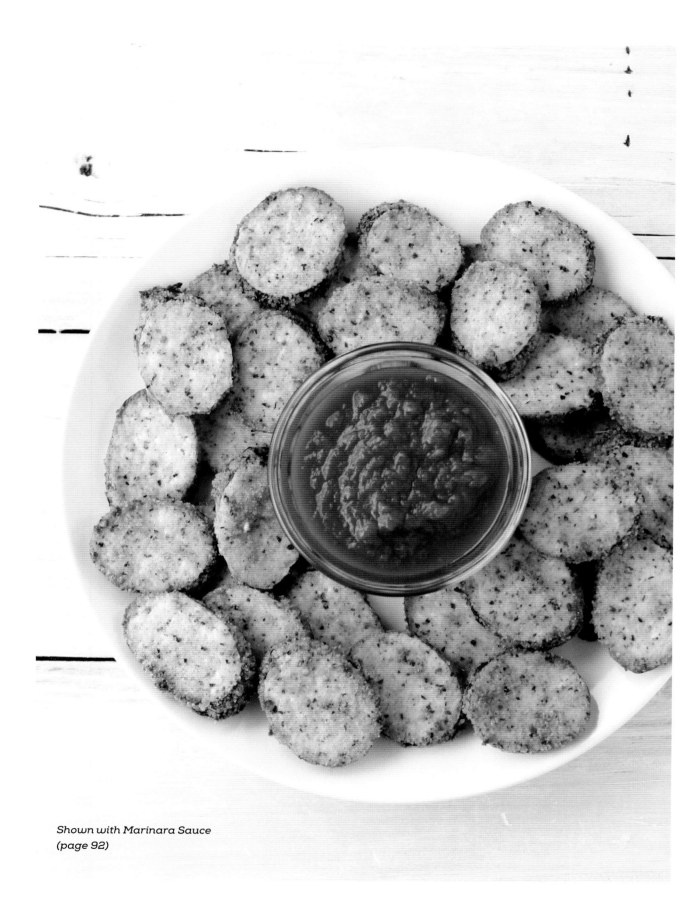

*Shown with Marinara Sauce
(page 92)*

BREADED ZUCCHINI CHIPS

• MAKES 4 SERVINGS •

At the peak of summer, when zucchini are plentiful, you can feel like they're coming out your ears. Steamed zucchini, grilled zucchini, zucchini bread. . . . But with this recipe, you'll forget you're eating yet more zucchini, or even a vegetable. Pair them with a warm Marinara Sauce (page 92) for a real treat.

1 cup (118 g) GF bread crumbs (see opposite to make your own)

2 tablespoons grated Parmesan cheese

½ teaspoon dried oregano

½ teaspoon dried basil

¼ teaspoon garlic powder

¼ teaspoon salt

¼ teaspoon pepper

1 egg

1 teaspoon water

2 zucchini, cut on a bias into ¼-inch (0.5 cm) slices

Olive oil

1. Preheat the oven to 400°F (200°C). Place a wire rack over a baking sheet and grease well with nonstick cooking spray or olive oil.

2. Combine the bread crumbs, Parmesan, oregano, basil, garlic powder, salt, and pepper in a wide, shallow bowl. Whisk together the egg and water in a separate wide, shallow bowl.*

3. Using one hand for the wet and one for the dry, dip each slice of zucchini in the egg, then in the bread crumb mixture, and place on the prepared wire rack. Repeat with the remaining slices of zucchini until all have been coated in bread crumbs. Use an olive oil mister to evenly and lightly coat the tops of the zucchini slices, just enough to moisten, but not saturate, the bread crumbs.

4. Bake for about 18 minutes, until the breading is brown and the zucchini is cooked through and tender.

*If you don't have an olive oil mister, adjust the breading procedure by following the egg-free instructions below.

Make your own . . .

GLUTEN-FREE BREAD CRUMBS: Start with slices of our Sandwich Bread (page 80) or store-bought gluten-free bread. Pulse in the food processor to make coarse crumbs. Spread in a thin layer on a baking sheet and bake at 350°F (175°C) for 10 minutes, watching carefully, until dried out. Pulse again in the processor to make fine crumbs. (Gluten-free crackers or cereal can also make easy bread crumbs, without needing to be dried in the oven.)

NOTE: The *refined-sugar-free*, *dairy/lactose/casein-free*, *egg-free*, and *corn-free* statuses of this recipe are partially dependent on the ingredients in your bread crumbs. Our Sandwich Bread (page 80) can be made any combination of the above.

KIDS CAN . . .

✳ Collect ingredients from the pantry and refrigerator

✳ Measure dry ingredients

✳ Dump dry ingredients into a bowl

✳ Mix dry ingredients with a whisk, spoon, or fork

✳ Crack the egg and make the egg wash

✳ Bread the zucchini slices

✳ Mist the breaded zucchini slices with olive oil

To make this recipe . . . .

EGG-FREE
- Make sure you're using egg-free bread crumbs.
- Omit the egg wash and replace with 3 tablespoons olive oil. Dip each zucchini slice in the olive oil, coat with bread crumbs, and transfer to the wire rack. Omit misting with olive oil.

DAIRY/LACTOSE/CASEIN-FREE
- Omit the Parmesan cheese.
- Check the ingredients of your bread crumbs.

VEGAN
- Use the dairy-free and egg-free substitutions.

SWEET POTATER TOTS

• MAKES ABOUT 40 TOTS •

Bite-size Tater Tots, that classic from Ore-Ida, are a favorite of kids everywhere, and a school lunch-room staple. These sweet potater tots (we're suckers for a good play on words) swap in more-nutritious sweet potatoes for the traditional white potatoes.

2 pounds (907 g) whole, unpeeled sweet potatoes (about 3 medium)
3 tablespoons Artisan GF Flour Blend (page 27)
1 teaspoon salt
1½ to 2 quarts (1½ to 2 liters) oil, for frying

1. Bring a large pot of water to a boil. Place the whole sweet potatoes into the pot and boil for 15 minutes, until they are fork-tender but not soft. When cool enough to handle, peel the skin off and shred the potatoes using a large-holed grater. Wrap in a kitchen towel, nut bag (usually used for squeezing nut milk out of nut pulp), or paper towels and squeeze out as much moisture as possible. (Since paper towels can tear, it is easier to use cloth, but note that it will stain.)

2. In a bowl, combine the dried shredded sweet potato, flour, and salt. Toss to combine and coat evenly. Pinch off about 1 tablespoon of potato and press into a cylinder shape in your hand, then flatten each end to make the traditional Tater Tot shape. Repeat to make about 40 tots.

3. Meanwhile, heat the oil to 350°F (175°C) in a large (at least 4-quart/4-liter) saucepot. Fry the tots in batches, without crowding, for about 5 minutes, until golden brown. Remove from the oil with a slotted spoon and drain on paper towels or a brown paper bag.

KIDS CAN . . .

* Collect ingredients from the pantry and refrigerator

* Place sweet potatoes in pot of water (carefully)

* Peel and shred sweet potatoes

* Squeeze moisture out of sweet potatoes

* Add ingredients to bowl

* Mix ingredients

* Shape the tots

To **make this recipe** . . . .

CORN-FREE
• Use arrowroot flour to make a corn-free version of the Artisan GF Flour Blend (page 26).

GRAIN-FREE
• Substitute tapioca or potato starch for the flour blend.

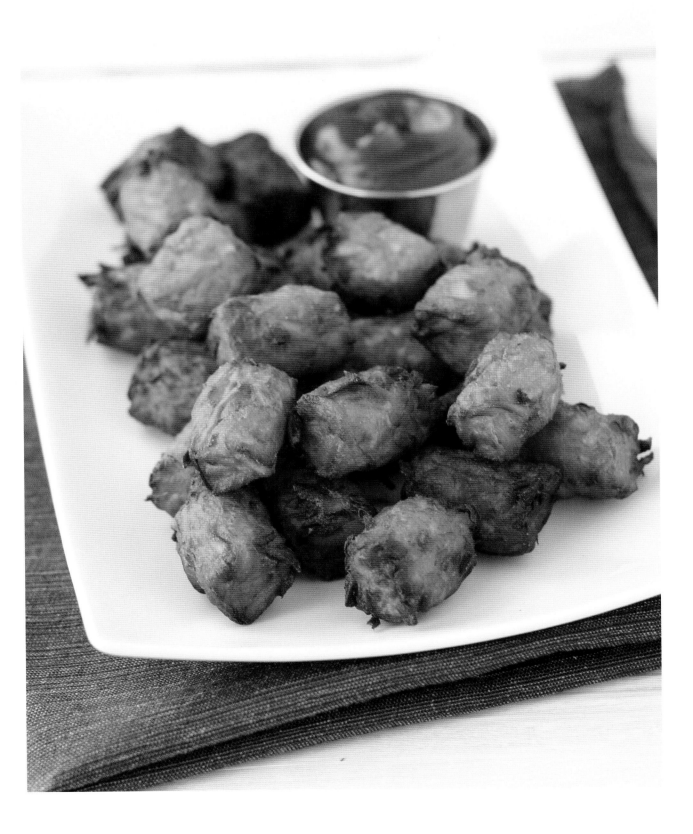

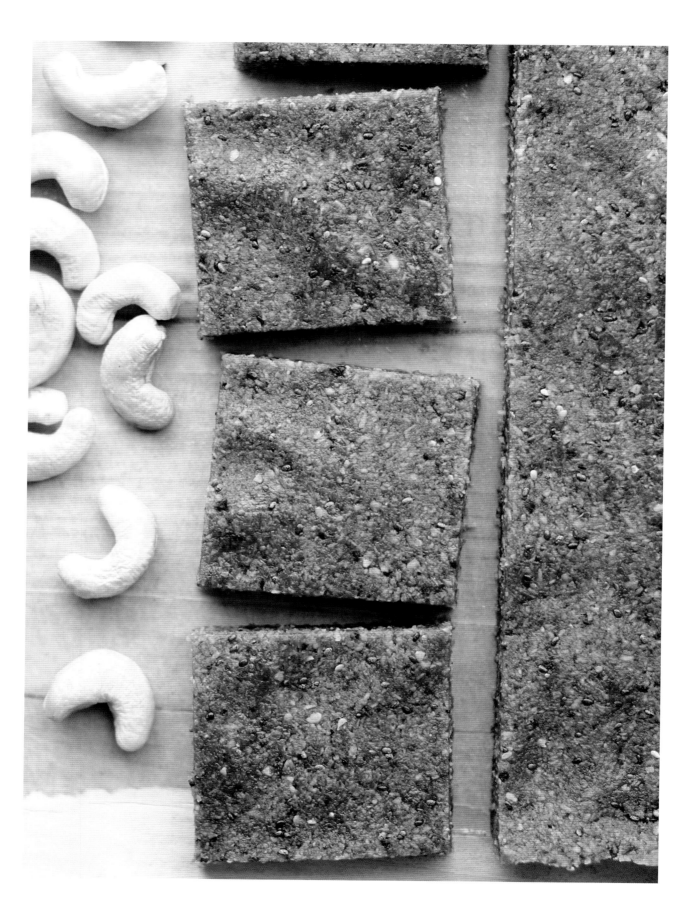

CASHEW COCONUT CHIA SQUARES

You can feel confident while handing out seconds that these snacks are a nutritional powerhouse. They are packed with protein and fiber and are also a great source of magnesium and potassium.

2 cups (160 g) unsweetened dehydrated shredded coconut

1½ cups (220 g) raw cashew pieces

10 dried figs, stems removed

¼ cup (60 ml) water

2 teaspoons GF pure vanilla extract

1 teaspoon ground cinnamon

¼ teaspoon salt

1 tablespoon chia seeds

1 tablespoon sesame seeds

1. Toast the shredded coconut in a dry large skillet over medium-high heat, stirring constantly, for 4 to 5 minutes, until golden brown. Set aside.

2. Place the cashew pieces in a food processor and process until they turn into a smooth cashew butter, 1 to 2 minutes. Add the figs, water, vanilla, cinnamon, and salt and process until smooth. Add the toasted coconut and the chia and sesame seeds and pulse to combine.

3. Line the bottom and sides of an 8 x 8-inch (20 x 20 cm) baking pan with parchment paper. Press the mixture into the prepared pan to form a uniform layer. Refrigerate for at least 1 hour to chill. Cut into 16 squares and serve. Refrigerate any uneaten squares for up to 1 week.

KIDS CAN . . .

* Collect ingredients from the pantry

* Count figs

* Measure ingredients

* Dump ingredients into the food processor

* Push the food processor buttons

* Press mixture into the pan

SANDWICH BREAD

• MAKES ONE 8½ X 4½-INCH (22 X 12 CM) LOAF •

In a gluten-free home it is critical to have great sandwich bread; this loaf is a weekly staple for our family. It can be sliced thin when cool, has a great crumb, and is fantastic for making traditional sandwiches, Grilled Cheese (page 111), and French Toast Sticks (page 35). It's also delicious hot out of the oven with a bit of jam or butter.

1½ cups (355 ml) warm water (about 115°F/45°C)

2 tablespoons sugar

2¼ teaspoons (1 packet) yeast

½ cup (35 g) milk powder

1 tablespoon butter, melted

3 eggs

3 cups (375 g) Artisan GF Flour Blend (page 27)

½ teaspoon xanthan gum

1½ teaspoons salt

KIDS CAN . . .

* Collect ingredients from the pantry and refrigerator

* Measure ingredients

* Dump ingredients into the mixing bowl

* Crack the eggs

* Stir the wet and dry ingredients together

* Grease the loaf pan

* Transfer the batter to the pan and smooth the top

1. Combine the water, sugar, and yeast in a bowl and allow to rest for 5 minutes, until the yeast is active and the mixture bubbly with a layer of foam on top.

2. Whisk the milk powder into the yeast mixture. Add the melted butter and whisk to combine. Whisk in the eggs. In a separate bowl, whisk together the flour, xanthan gum, and salt. Add the egg mixture to the flour mixture and mix with a spoon until smooth.

3. Grease an 8½ x 4½-inch (22 x 12 cm) loaf pan, including the top edge, with nonstick cooking spray or butter. Transfer the bread batter to the greased pan and smooth the top of the loaf with a wet spatula. Place in a warm location and allow to rise until the mixture is mounded over the top of the pan, 30 to 60 minutes.

4. Preheat the oven to 400°F (200°C).

5. Bake the bread for 30 minutes, until browned on top and with an internal temperature of 200°F (90°C to 95°C). Turn the loaf out of the pan and cool completely on a wire rack.

NOTE: To freeze, let the loaf cool completely and slice while still fresh. Lay the slices flat, placing parchment paper between layers of slices to prevent them from freezing together. Store in the freezer in a zip-top bag or airtight container.

To make this recipe . . . .

EGG-FREE

* In a small bowl, combine 3 tablespoons ground flaxseeds and ½ cup plus 1 tablespoon (135 ml) water. Allow the mixture to set for at least 2 minutes and use in place of the eggs.

DAIRY/LACTOSE/CASEIN-FREE

* Substitute 6 tablespoons (35 g) soy milk powder for the milk powder (note this introduces soy).

* Substitute vegan shortening for the butter.

CORN-FREE

* Use arrowroot flour to make a corn-free version of the Artisan GF Flour Blend (page 26).

REFINED-SUGAR-FREE

* Use 2 tablespoons honey instead of sugar.

VEGAN

* Use the dairy-free and egg-free substitutions.

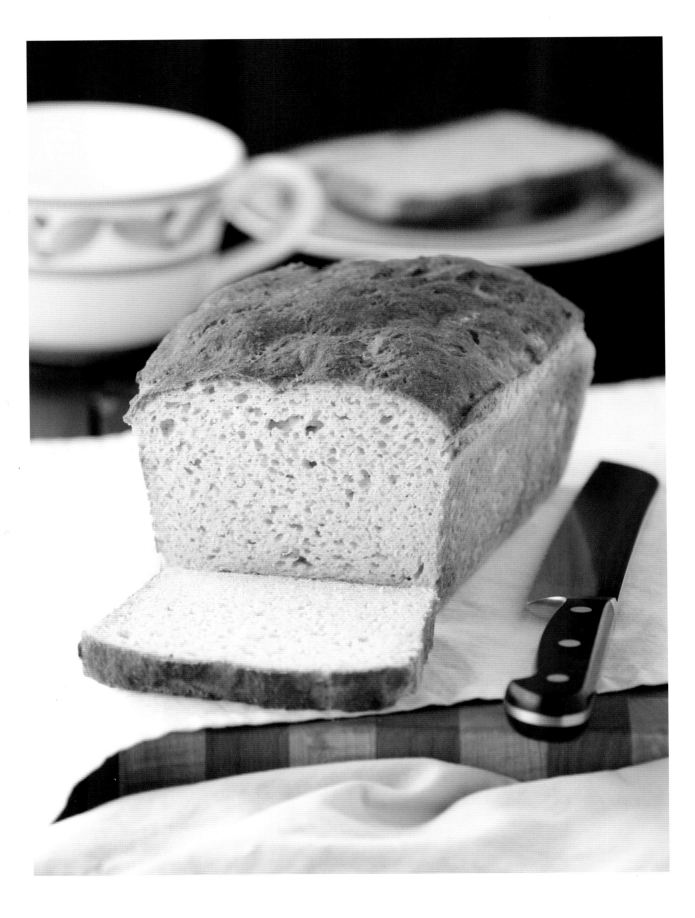

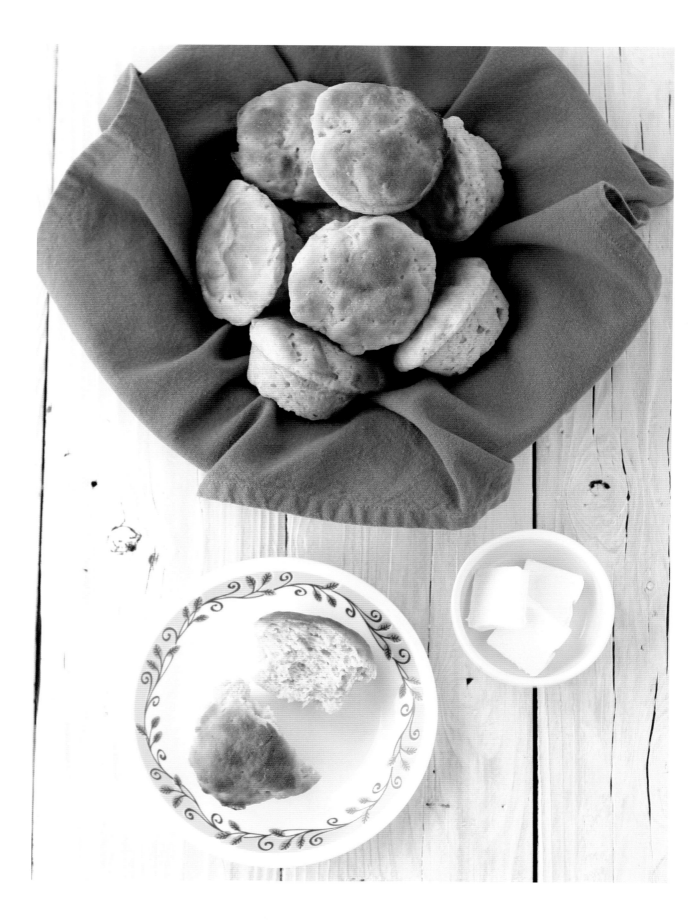

DINNER ROLLS

• MAKES 12 ROLLS •

These dinner rolls are golden brown and moist, with just the right amount of chewiness. We enjoy them by themselves, with a pat of butter, dipped in Slow Cooker Chicken Noodle Soup (page 127), or even as mini sandwiches. Freeze any extras to defrost later and reheat to make like new.

¼ cup (60 ml) warm water (about 115°F/45°C)

1 teaspoon sugar

2¼ teaspoons (1 packet) yeast

¾ cup (180 ml) milk

¼ cup (85 g) honey

1 teaspoon salt

½ cup (1 stick) butter

3 eggs

2¾ cups (344 g) Artisan GF Flour Blend (page 27)

½ teaspoon xanthan gum

1. Combine the water, sugar, and yeast in a bowl and allow to rest for 5 minutes, until the yeast is active and the mixture bubbly with a layer of foam on top.

2. In a saucepan, heat the milk, honey, salt, and ⅓ cup of the butter over medium-low heat (115°F to 120°F/45°C) to melt the butter.

3. While the milk mixture is heating, use 1 tablespoon of the butter to grease the cups of a 12-cup muffin tin, including the top rim of each cup.

4. Remove the milk mixture from the heat and whisk in the eggs. Whisk in the yeast mixture. In a separate bowl, whisk together the flour and xanthan gum, then whisk it into the yeast-milk mixture.

5. Divide the batter among the 12 muffin cups and smooth the tops gently with wet fingers. Cover with an inverted pan or container and let rise in a warm place for 45 minutes.

6. Preheat the oven to 475°F (245°C).

7. Melt the remaining butter. Bake the rolls for 5 minutes. Open the oven and use a pastry brush to brush the melted butter on top of the rolls. Turn the oven down to 350°F (175°C) and bake for an additional 8 minutes, until the rolls are deep golden brown on top. Remove from the oven and take the rolls out of the pan as soon as you can handle them. Cool on a wire rack.

NOTE: To reheat, pop in a 350°F (175°C) oven until warm, or microwave (times vary based on microwave strength; watch carefully).

KIDS CAN . . .

* Collect ingredients from the pantry and refrigerator
* Measure ingredients
* Crack the eggs
* Dump ingredients into the saucepan and mixing bowl
* Stir the ingredients together
* Grease the muffin tin
* Divide the dough among the muffin cups and help smooth the tops

To make this recipe . . . .

EGG-FREE
* In a small bowl, combine 3 tablespoons ground flaxseeds and ½ cup plus 1 tablespoon (135 ml) water. Allow the mixture to set for at least 2 minutes and use in place of the eggs.

DAIRY/LACTOSE/CASEIN-FREE
* Substitute almond milk (or, for nut allergies, rice or hemp milk) for the cow's milk.
* Substitute ⅓ cup vegan shortening for the butter in the rolls and to grease the muffin tin.
* Do not brush anything on the rolls as they bake.
* Cover the rolls with aluminum foil if they begin to brown too much while baking.

CORN-FREE
* Use arrowroot flour to make a corn-free version of the Artisan GF Flour Blend (page 26).

REFINED-SUGAR-FREE
* Substitute honey for the sugar used to activate the yeast.

VEGAN
* Use the dairy-free and egg-free substitutions.

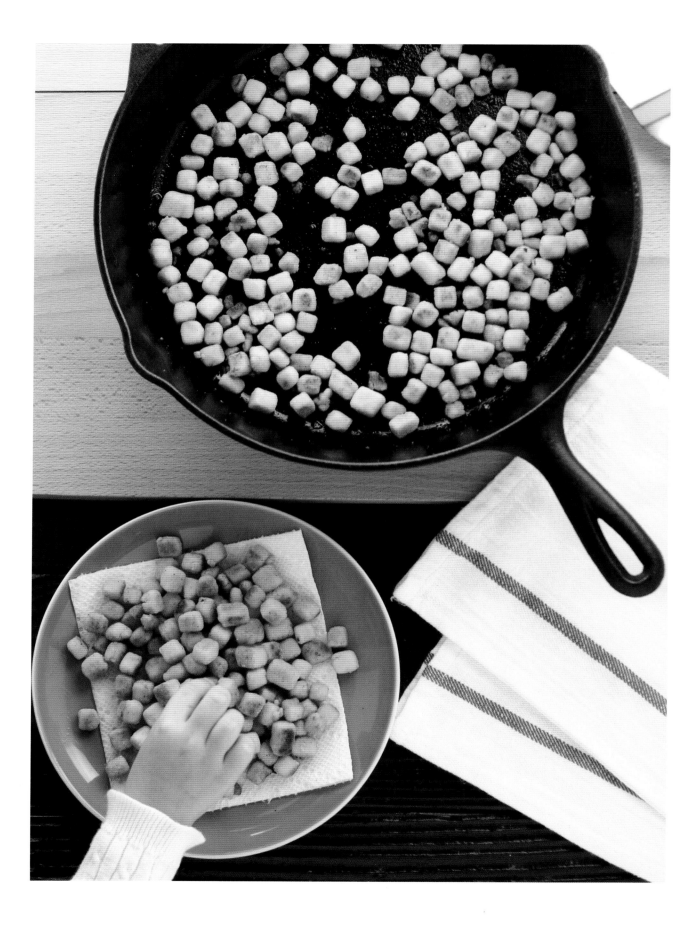

TOFU POPCORN

• MAKES 3 TO 5 SERVINGS •

Tofu popcorn could make a tofu fan out of anyone, kids included. Pan-fried, their golden-brown, slightly crispy exterior and silky smooth interior make them nosh-able on their own as a snack, the star protein on a dinner plate, or a protein substitute in other dishes, such as for chicken in a stir-fry.

1¼ cups (156 g) Artisan GF Flour Blend (page 27)

1¼ teaspoons garlic powder

1¼ teaspoons salt

14 ounces (397 g) extra-firm tofu, drained, patted dry, and cut into small cubes

½ cup (120 ml) olive oil, divided

KIDS CAN...

* Collect ingredients from the pantry and refrigerator

* Measure dry ingredients

* Dump dry ingredients into mixing bowl

* Mix dry ingredients with a whisk, spoon, or fork

* Cut the tofu into cubes with an age-appropriate knife

* Toss the tofu cubes in the flour

* Shake the colander

1. In a large bowl, combine the flour, garlic powder, and salt. Add half of the tofu and toss to coat all sides of the cubes. Transfer to a colander with large holes. Tap over the bowl or your garbage to remove any excess flour.

2. Heat ¼ cup of the olive oil in a large skillet over medium-high heat. Add the floured tofu cubes and sauté, turning regularly, until golden brown on all sides, 10 to 12 minutes. Remove from the pan and drain in a bowl lined with a paper towel.

3. Heat the remaining ¼ cup olive oil in the pan and flour and fry the remaining tofu pieces.

To make this recipe ....

CORN-FREE
* Use arrowroot flour to make a corn-free version of the Artisan GF Flour Blend (page 26).

GRAIN-FREE
* Substitute tapioca or potato starch for the flour blend.

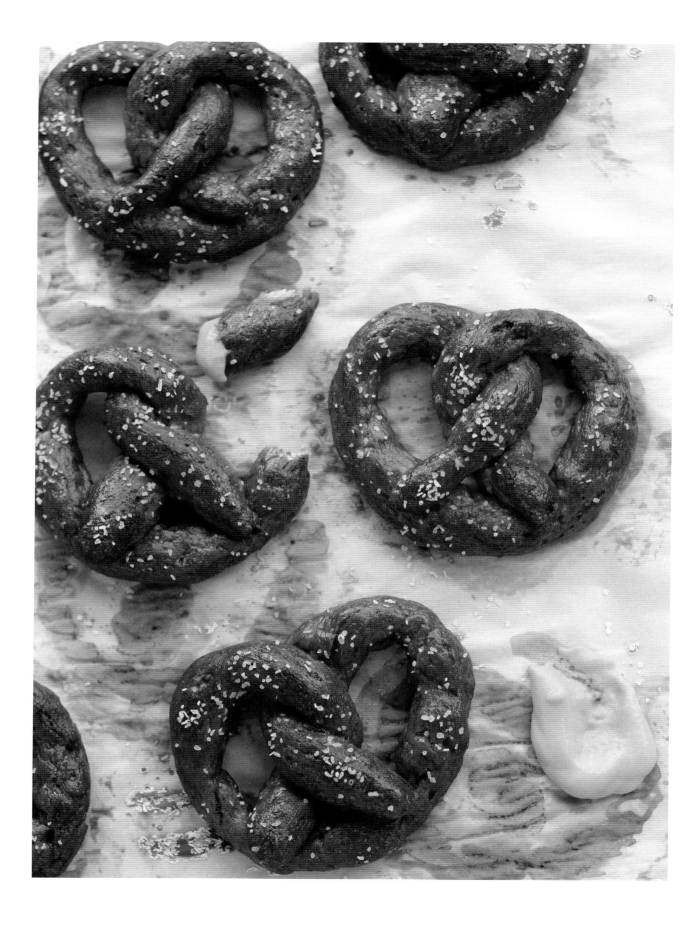

SOFT PRETZELS

• MAKES 16 PRETZELS •

Whether watching Major League Baseball on TV or Little League in person, you can still have an authentic ballpark pretzel experience! These are the real deal, boiled in baking soda water to provide the traditional pretzel taste, texture, and browning. They're best hot out of the oven but also freeze well.

1½ cups (355 ml) warm water (115°F/45°C)

1 tablespoon sugar

2¼ teaspoons (1 packet) yeast

¼ cup (½ stick, 56 g) butter, melted

4 egg yolks

3½ cups (438 g) Artisan GF Flour Blend (page 27)

2 teaspoons xanthan gum

1½ teaspoons salt

8 cups (1.9 liters) water

½ cup (118 g) baking soda

1 egg

Kosher salt

1. Combine the water, sugar, and yeast in a bowl and allow to rest for 5 minutes, until the yeast is active and the mixture bubbly with a layer of foam on top. Add the butter and egg yolks and whisk to combine.

2. In a separate bowl, whisk together the flour, xanthan gum, and salt. Stir in the yeast mixture to form a slightly sticky dough.

3. Line two baking sheets with parchment paper. Divide the dough into 16 equal pieces. If the dough is sticky, lightly coat your hands with olive oil to work with the dough.

4. Roll one piece into a snake-like roll that is 18 inches (45 cm) long. Form the snake into a big upside-down letter "U." About one-third of the way from the open end of the U, cross the tails twice. Then flip the tails up so that they just cross the loop and press lightly so the pretzel holds its shape. Repeat to make 16 pretzels.

5. Place the pretzels on the prepared baking sheets. Place the baking sheets in a warm location and allow the pretzels to rise for 1 hour.

6. Near the end of the rise, preheat the oven to 400°F (200°C). Combine the water and baking soda in a wide-bottomed saucepan and bring to a boil.

7. Bake the pretzels for 4 minutes. Remove the baking sheets from the oven.

8. Boil the pretzels in batches (each with a single floating layer of pretzels) in the baking soda water for 45 seconds per side (1 minute 30 seconds total), carefully flipping to prevent breakage. Remove with a slotted spoon and return to the parchment-lined baking sheets.

9. Whisk the egg in a small bowl. Use a pastry brush to coat the tops and sides of each pretzel with the egg. Sprinkle lightly with the kosher salt.

10. Return to the oven and bake the pretzels for another 18 minutes, until golden and cooked through.

(RECIPE CONTINUES)

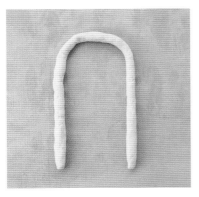
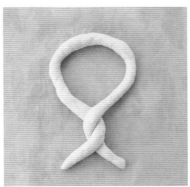
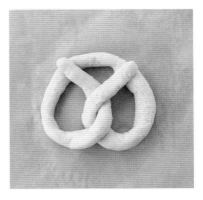

* Collect ingredients from the pantry and refrigerator

* Measure ingredients

* Dump ingredients into mixing bowl

* Stir the ingredients together

* Roll the divided dough into snakes and shape

* Sprinkle salt on the parboiled pretzels

VARIATION

PRETZEL BITES: You can also make this recipe into tasty pretzel bites. Simply roll the dough into a long snake and cut into 1- to 2-inch (2.5 to 5 cm) pieces. Then follow steps 4 through 6 and finish baking in the oven for 12 to 14 minutes.

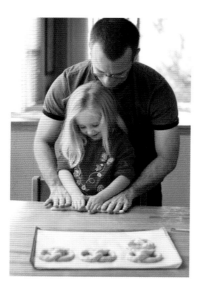 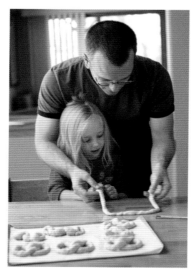 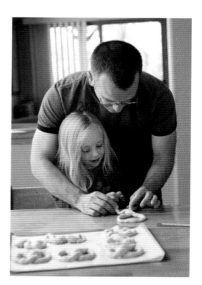

To make this recipe . . . .

EGG-FREE
* Omit the egg yolks.
* Sprinkle the salt directly onto the boiled pretzels without the egg wash.

DAIRY/LACTOSE/CASEIN-FREE
* Substitute vegan shortening for the butter.

CORN-FREE
* Use arrowroot flour to make a corn-free version of the Artisan GF Flour Blend (page 26).

REFINED-SUGAR-FREE
* Substitute honey for the sugar to activate the yeast.

VEGAN
* Use the dairy-free and egg-free substitutions.

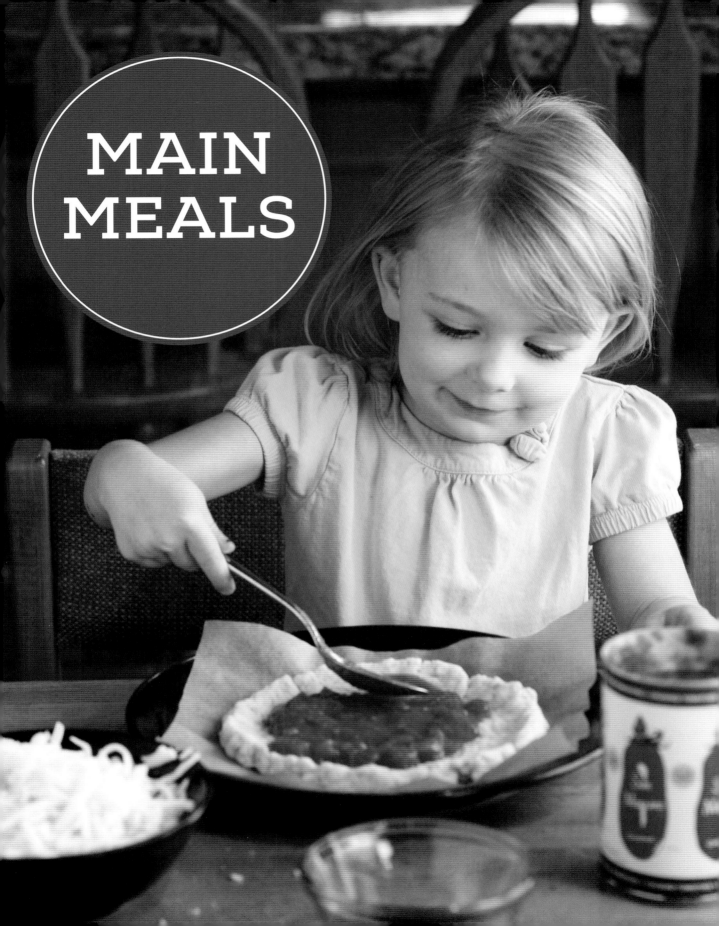

MAIN MEALS

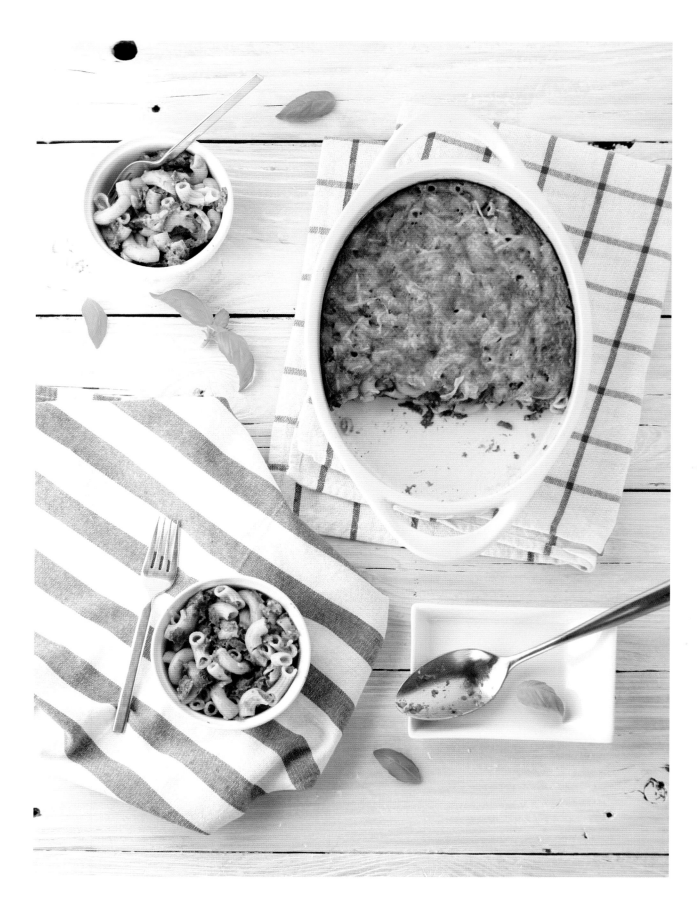

PESTO MAC AND CHEESE

• MAKES ONE 9 X 9-INCH PAN OR 2-QUART CASSEROLE •

This dish combines a traditional from-scratch macaroni and cheese with a healthful pesto, made with spinach in addition to the usual basil. The result is a green mac and cheese that's not super cheesy yet loses none of the richness and flavor of the original.

8 ounces (227 g) short GF pasta
   (e.g., elbow macaroni)

2 cups (90 g) packed spinach leaves

½ cup (18 g) fresh basil leaves

¼ cup (37 g) raw cashew pieces

4 ounces (113 g) sharp cheddar cheese, cut into cubes

¼ cup (23 g) plus 2 tablespoons grated Parmesan cheese

1 garlic clove, peeled

1 cup (240 ml) milk

1 egg

Salt and pepper

1. Preheat the oven to 375°F (190°C). Grease a 9 x 9-inch (23 x 23 cm) baking pan or 2-quart (1.9 L) casserole with nonstick cooking spray or olive oil.

2. Bring a large pot of salted water to a boil. Add the pasta and cook until al dente. Drain.

3. Meanwhile, combine the spinach, basil, cashews, cheddar, ¼ cup of the Parmesan, and garlic in the food processor and process until a paste forms. Scrape down the sides of the bowl and add ¾ cup milk. Blend until the mixture is smooth. Add the remaining milk, the egg, and a dash each of salt and pepper and process until incorporated.

4. In a large bowl, mix the cooked pasta with the spinach mixture. Pour into the prepared pan. Top with the remaining 2 tablespoons grated Parmesan. Bake for 30 minutes, until the top is lightly browned and the pasta is set.

VARIATION

PESTO MACARONI: Omit the cheddar, Parmesan, milk, and egg. Toss the spinach mixture with the hot cooked and drained noodles, but do not bake

KIDS CAN . . .

* Collect ingredients from the pantry and refrigerator

* Measure ingredients

* Dump ingredients into the food processor

* Press the food processor buttons

* Crack the egg

* Mix the pasta and spinach mixture together with a spoon

To make this recipe . . . .

TREE-NUT-FREE
● Substitute hemp seeds for the cashew pieces.

EGG-FREE, DAIRY-FREE, AND VEGAN
● Follow the instructions to make the Pesto Macaroni variation.

CORN-FREE
● Make sure you're using a corn-free pasta, such as one made from brown rice or quinoa.

SPAGHETTI SQUASH "PASTA" WITH EASY MARINARA SAUCE

• MAKES 4 SERVINGS •

If you're looking for an alternative to traditional spaghetti noodles, spaghetti squash lives up to its name. Oven-roasting the squash brings out its flavors, which can stand on their own or pair well with our marinara recipe or your favorite pasta sauce.

SPAGHETTI SQUASH

One 3-pound (1.25 to 1.5 kg) spaghetti squash

2 tablespoons olive oil

½ teaspoon garlic powder

½ teaspoon dried basil

½ teaspoon dried oregano

½ teaspoon salt

½ teaspoon pepper

MARINARA SAUCE

1 tablespoon olive oil

½ medium onion, diced

2 garlic cloves, grated or minced

1 teaspoon dried basil

1 teaspoon dried oregano

1½ cups (411 g) diced tomatoes or one 14.5-ounce (411 g) can no-salt-added diced tomatoes

One 6-ounce (170 g) can tomato paste

1 tablespoon balsamic vinegar

1. To roast the squash: Preheat the oven to 375°F (190°C).

2. Cut the spaghetti squash in half lengthwise using a large knife and scoop out the seeds. Place the squash cut-side *up* in a baking pan and coat each half with the olive oil, ensuring all of the squash flesh is covered. Sprinkle the garlic powder, basil, oregano, salt, and pepper evenly over the halves. Roast for 50 to 60 minutes,* until the squash is very tender when poked with a fork, basting every 20 minutes with the liquid that accumulates in the scooped out portion of the squash "bowl." You may drizzle with extra olive oil if your squash seems dry and the "bowls" don't have enough basting liquid.

3. Cool the squash for 10 minutes, then scoop out the flesh and tease apart the fibers to create the "spaghetti."

4. To make the marinara sauce: Heat the olive oil in a medium saucepan over medium heat. Add the onion and garlic and sauté until soft and fragrant, about 2 minutes. Add the basil and oregano and sauté for another minute. Add the tomatoes and simmer over medium heat for about 5 minutes. Puree the sauce with a handheld immersion blender to your desired level of smoothness or chunkiness. Stir in the tomato paste and balsamic vinegar and cook another 5 minutes.

*A larger squash will take longer to become tender.

KIDS CAN...

* Collect ingredients from the pantry and refrigerator

* Measure ingredients

* Coat squash halves with olive oil

* Sprinkle seasonings over squash

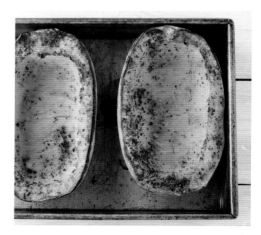

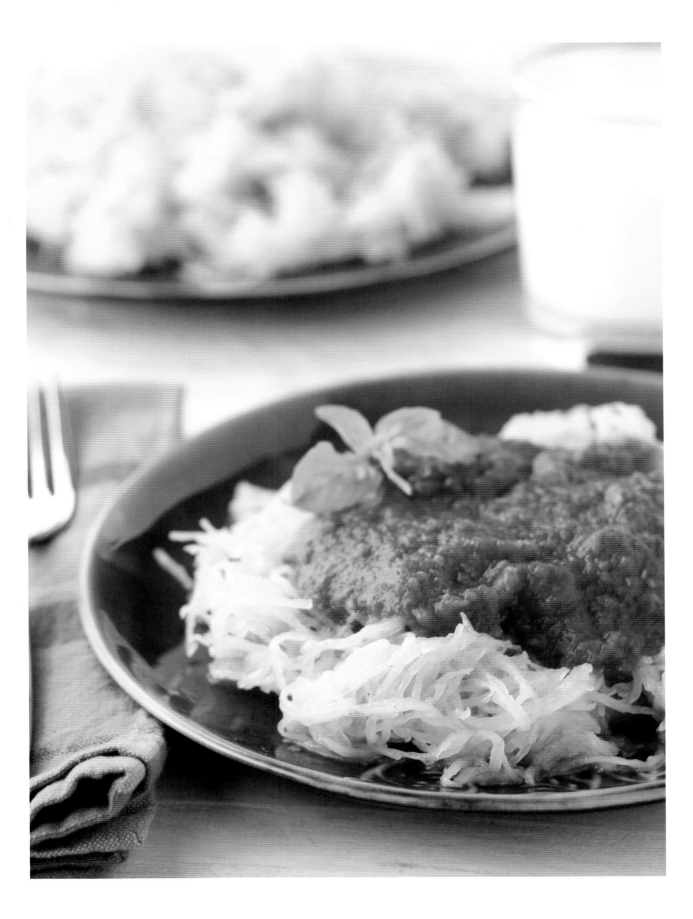

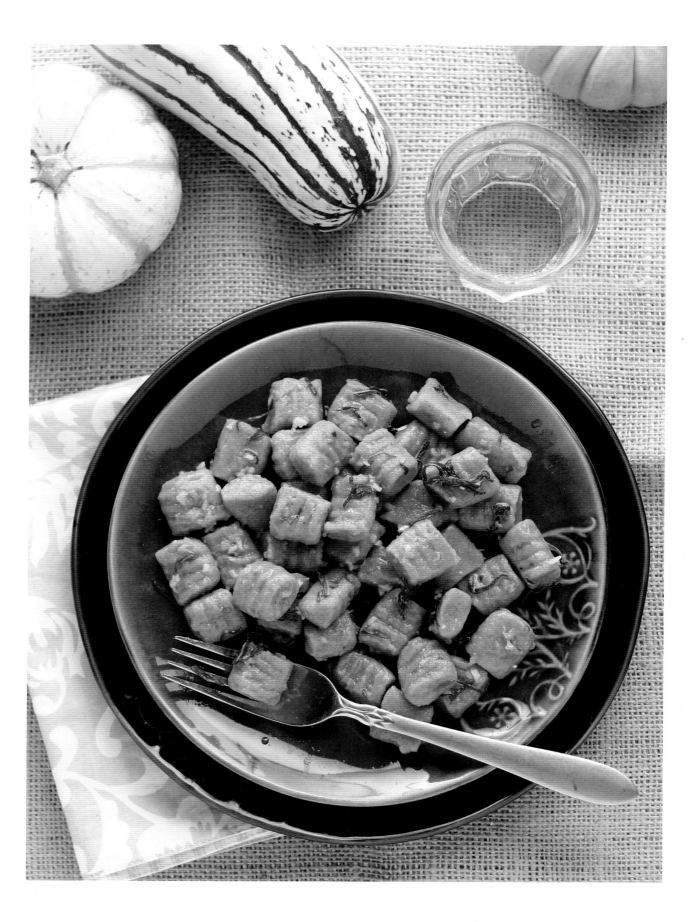

PUMPKIN GNOCCHI NUGGETS

• MAKES 6 SERVINGS •

Kids tend to love chicken nuggets, so why not gnocchi nuggets? Gnocchi are a hybrid of pasta and dumplings, usually made with flour and potato. In this case, the flour is gluten-free and we've swapped in pumpkin for the potato, paired the gnocchi with a simple sage–brown butter sauce, and given the dish a cute, kid-friendly name. Making them is a job ripe for little hands, which can then help devour these nuggets later for dinner.

GNOCCHI NUGGETS

2 cups (425 g) pureed roasted pumpkin, or one 15-ounce (425 g) can pumpkin puree

2 eggs, beaten

¼ cup grated Parmesan cheese, plus more for serving, optional

¼ teaspoon ground nutmeg

¼ teaspoon garlic powder

1 teaspoon salt

¼ teaspoon pepper

2½ to 3 cups (313 to 375 g) Artisan GF Flour Blend (page 27)

SAGE BUTTER SAUCE

¼ cup (½ stick, 56 g) butter

10 large sage leaves, chiffonade (sliced into long, thin strips)

2 garlic cloves, grated or minced

KIDS CAN . . .

* Collect ingredients from the pantry and refrigerator

* Measure ingredients

* Dump ingredients into mixing bowl

* Mix ingredients with a spoon or whisk

* Cut the snakes of dough into gnocchi nuggets with a butter knife

* Roll the gnocchi over the fork tines

1. To make the gnocchi: In a large bowl, combine the pumpkin, eggs, cheese, nutmeg, garlic powder, salt, and pepper and mix until smooth. Add 2½ cups flour and mix to form a soft dough. If the dough is sticky, add additional flour a little at a time, up to 3 cups total. The moisture content of roasted and canned pumpkin can vary widely, which affects the stickiness of the dough.

2. Divide the dough into 4 equal pieces. Roll one piece into a snake-like roll about ½ inch (1.25 cm) in diameter. The dough will be tender. Cut the snake into ¾-inch (2 cm) segments and roll each segment over the tines of a fork to create grooves (these not only look fancy, but also help your gnocchi hold more sauce!). Set the completed gnocchi aside on a baking sheet and sprinkle lightly with flour to prevent them from sticking together. Repeat with the remaining dough.

3. Bring a large pot of salted water to a boil. Add the gnocchi in batches (each with an uncrowded floating single layer). When you initially drop them in the water, they will sink. Once they float, let them continue to cook for 2 to 3 minutes. Remove from the water with a slotted spoon and place in a colander to allow any excess water to drain.

4. To make the sauce, heat the butter, sage, and garlic in a large skillet over medium heat until the butter is foamy and then turns golden brown, 1 to 2 minutes. Remove from the heat. Add the gnocchi to the butter sauce and toss to coat. Serve warm with additional Parmesan cheese if desired.

To make this recipe . . . .

DAIRY/LACTOSE/CASEIN-FREE
* Omit the Parmesan cheese.
* Substitute olive oil for the butter.

CORN-FREE
* Use arrowroot flour to make a corn-free version of the Artisan GF Flour Blend (page 26).

PERSONAL PIZZAS

• MAKES 6 INDIVIDUAL PIZZAS •

What kid doesn't like a good pizza? By creating personal pizzas, your children can load them up with toppings themselves and enjoy the fruits of their labor. This is a fun activity for a children's birthday party. You can also bake a batch (or several) of the untopped pizza crusts and pop them in the freezer, so they're ready to go anytime your family is craving a fresh-baked pizza.

1½ cups (355 ml) warm water (about 115°F/45°C)

2 tablespoons sugar

4½ teaspoons (2 packets) yeast

2¾ cups plus 1 tablespoon (350 g) Artisan GF Flour Blend (page 27)

2 teaspoons xanthan gum

1½ teaspoons salt

3 tablespoons olive oil

One 14.5-ounce (411 g) can San Marzano tomatoes, crushed or pureed (1¾ cups)

8 ounces (227 g) mozzarella cheese, shredded

Dried oregano

Dried basil

OPTIONAL TOPPINGS

Pepperoni

Browned sausage

Diced pepper

Diced onion

Sliced mushrooms

Sliced olives

Fresh basil

KIDS CAN . . .

* Collect ingredients from the pantry and refrigerator

* Measure ingredients

* Stir the ingredients together

* Shape and press pizza crusts

* Add toppings to pizzas

1. Preheat the oven to 400°F (205°C). Cut parchment paper into six 8-inch (20 cm) squares.

2. Combine the water, sugar, and yeast in a bowl and allow the mixture to rest for 5 minutes, until the yeast is active and the mixture bubbly with a layer of foam on top.

3. In a separate bowl, whisk together the flour, xanthan gum, and salt. Add 2 tablespoons olive oil to the yeast mixture, then pour it into the whisked flour. Mix to form a dough that is soft and slightly sticky to the touch. Drizzle the remaining 1 tablespoon olive oil on the dough and turn to coat the dough and your hands.

4. Divide the dough into 6 equal balls. Press each ball into individual pizzas about 6 inches (15 cm) in diameter, one on each piece of parchment paper. Make sure there is a small lip on the edge of each pizza crust to hold in the sauce and toppings. Transfer the pizzas-on-parchment onto 2 baking sheets. Bake the crusts for 8 minutes, until slightly golden on the edges. Remove from the oven and increase the oven temperature to 425°F (220°C).

5. Top the pizzas with the tomatoes, cheese, dried herbs, and desired toppings. Place the pizzas-on-parchment directly on the top oven rack (no pan), and bake for 12 to 15 minutes, until the crust and cheese are brown. Depending upon the size of your oven you may need to bake the pizzas in batches.

NOTE: This recipe can also be used to make two 12-inch (30 cm) pizzas or one 9 x 11-inch (23 x 28 cm) deep dish pizza. For either of these options, par-bake for 10 minutes.

VARIATION

You could also use the Potato Rolls (page 139) to make English muffin–style pizzas in the oven or toaster oven.

To make this recipe . . . .

DAIRY/LACTOSE/CASEIN-FREE
* Use nondairy cheese.

CORN-FREE
* Use arrowroot flour to make a corn-free version of the Artisan GF Flour Blend (page 26).

REFINED-SUGAR-FREE
* Substitute honey for the sugar used to activate the yeast.

VEGETARIAN
* Use only vegetarian toppings.

VEGAN
* Follow the instructions for both the dairy-free and vegetarian versions.

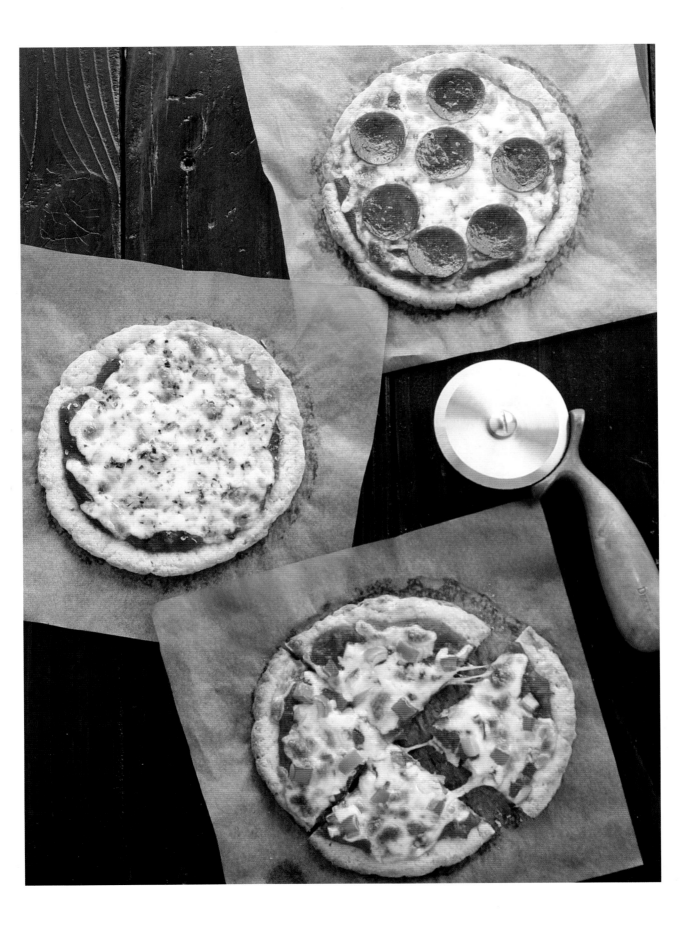

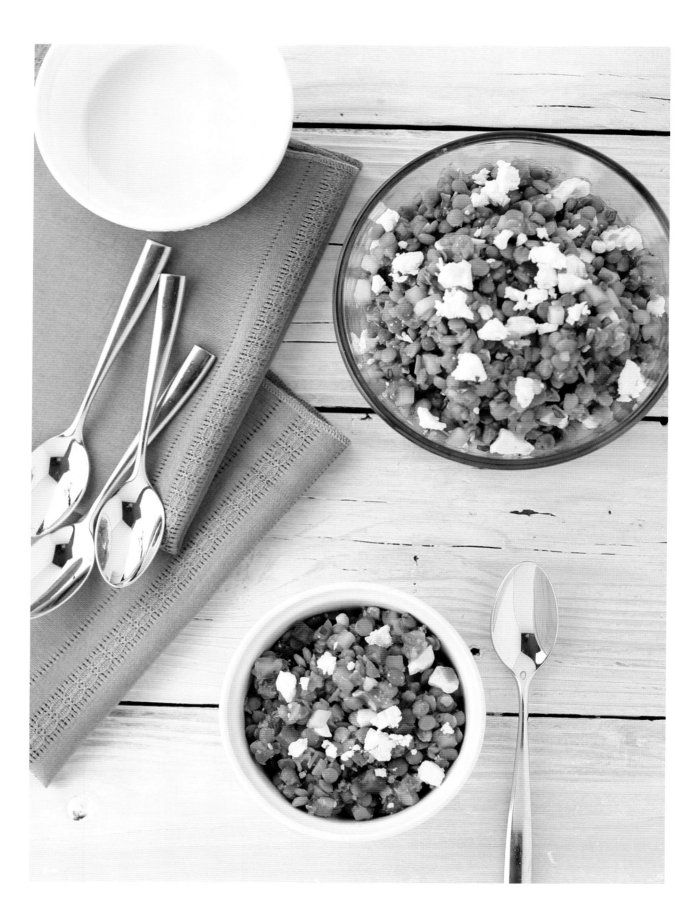

LENTIL SALAD

• MAKES 4 TO 6 SERVINGS •

Lentils are an all-star member of the legume family, full of fiber, protein, magnesium, and iron. Since lentils cook relatively quickly, this salad is a snap to prepare.

1 cup (190 g) brown or green lentils, rinsed in a fine-mesh strainer

2 cups (475 ml) water

2 garlic cloves, peeled

2 bay leaves

Salt

½ cucumber, peeled, seeded, and diced small (about ½ cup, 75 g)

1 medium tomato, diced small (about ½ cup, 105 g)

2 tablespoons chopped fresh basil

¼ cup (30 g) crumbled feta cheese, plus extra for garnish

Juice of 1 lemon (about ¼ cup/60 ml)

¼ cup (60 ml) olive oil

Pepper

1. Combine the rinsed lentils, water, garlic, and bay leaves in a saucepan. Bring to a boil over high heat. Turn the heat down and gently simmer, uncovered, for 20 to 30 minutes, until the lentils are tender. If needed, add additional water to keep the lentils covered while they simmer. Drain in a fine-mesh strainer, place in a bowl, and season with ½ teaspoon salt, tossing to incorporate while hot. Remove and discard the garlic cloves and bay leaves. Let cool.

2. Add the cucumber, tomato, basil, and feta to the lentils and toss to combine. In a small separate bowl, whisk together the lemon juice and olive oil. Drizzle over the lentils and toss to coat. Taste and season, if desired, with salt and pepper. Chill and serve. (The salad will keep for up to one week in the refrigerator.)

KIDS CAN . . .

* Collect ingredients from the pantry and refrigerator

* Measure ingredients

* Cut cucumber (after peeled and seeded) and tomato with age-appropriate knife

* Place ingredients into saucepan and mixing bowl

* Juice the lemon using a citrus reamer over a strainer to catch the seeds

* Whisk together the lemon and olive oil

* Mix all ingredients with a spoon

To make this recipe . . . .

DAIRY/LACTOSE/CASEIN-FREE
AND VEGAN
• Omit the cheese.

ASIAN QUINOA SALAD

• MAKES 4 SERVINGS •

This hearty salad is a marriage of East and West. It combines nutrition-packed quinoa, native to South America and high in iron, fiber, and magnesium, with East Asian flavors as well as edamame which, like quinoa, is a complete protein, making the salad a self-contained meal.

1 cup (176 g) quinoa, rinsed in a fine-mesh strainer

2 cups (475 ml) water

1 tablespoon grated ginger (1- to 2-inch/2.5 to 5 cm piece)

2 tablespoons GF tamari wheat-free low-sodium soy sauce or GF soy sauce

2 tablespoons rice vinegar

2 tablespoons olive oil

1 tablespoon freshly squeezed orange juice

2 teaspoons honey

1½ teaspoons sesame oil

1 cup (150 g) cooked shelled edamame (green soybeans)

½ red bell pepper, diced small

½ cup (23 g) cilantro, chopped

4 scallions, sliced thin

1. Combine the rinsed quinoa and water in a saucepan and bring to a boil. Reduce the heat, cover, and simmer for 15 to 20 minutes, until all of the liquid is absorbed. The quinoa should be translucent and soft but not mushy. Refrigerate until cooled.

2. To make the vinaigrette, combine the ginger, tamari, rice vinegar, olive oil, orange juice, honey, and sesame oil in a bowl and whisk to combine.

3. In a large bowl, combine the cooled quinoa, edamame, red pepper, cilantro, scallions, and vinaigrette and toss. Serve chilled.

KIDS CAN . . .

* Collect ingredients from the pantry and refrigerator

* Rinse quinoa and put in saucepan

* Measure ingredients

* Dump ingredients in mixing bowl

* Mix vinaigrette with whisk

* Squeeze the edamame from their pods if they aren't already shelled

* Mix all ingredients together with a spoon

To make this recipe . . . .

SOY-FREE
- Substitute coconut aminos for the soy sauce, or make your own soy-free "soy" sauce (see page 123).
- Omit the edamame.

VEGAN
- Substitute agave nectar for the honey.

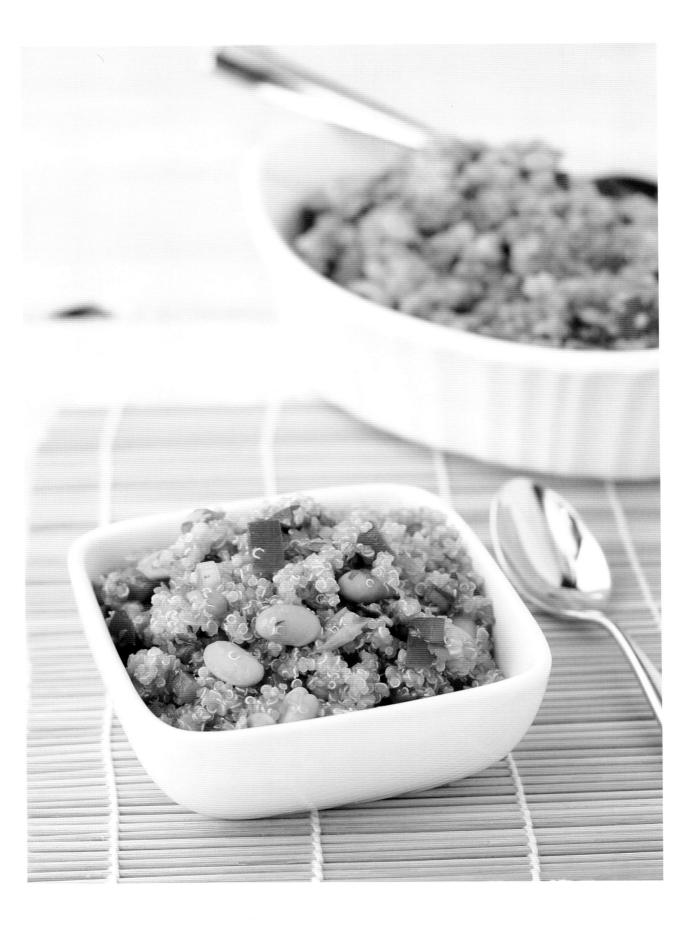

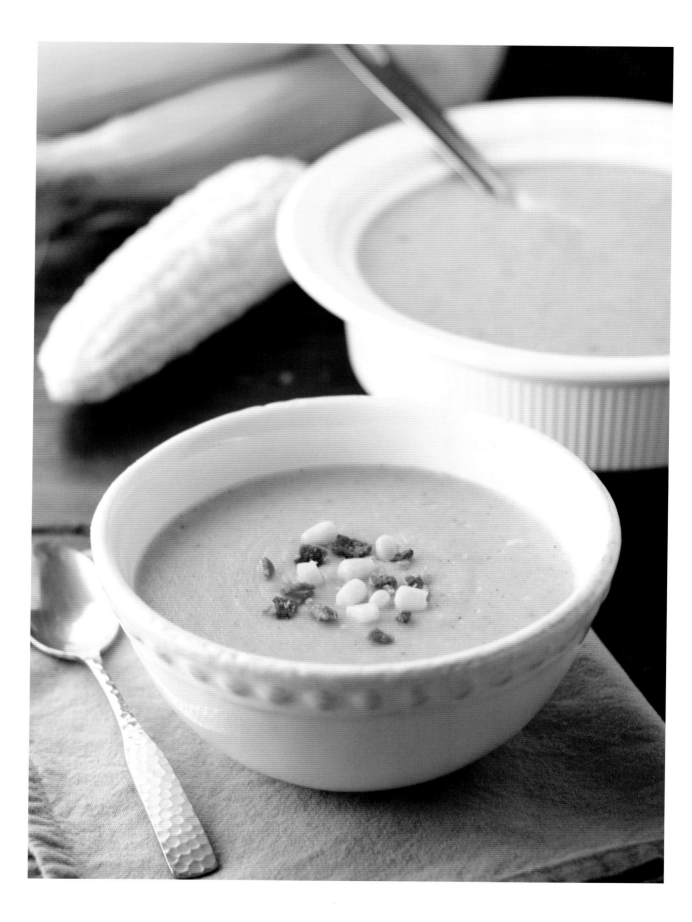

CORN CHOWDER

• MAKES 6 TO 8 SERVINGS •

Whether during corn's seasonal peak in summer when it's sweetest, or into the cooler months of fall and winter when we opt for the kernels from the freezer case, this simple chowder has a surprising twist: the addition of Swiss chard. It came about because our younger daughter, Charlotte, asked for a pink soup. We started with a creamy light-colored chowder and added something red—the Swiss chard. Alas, the chowder didn't turn pink, but our kids loved the end result anyway.

4 slices uncooked bacon

3 cups (454 g) corn kernels (from 6 ears, if using fresh)

1 large onion, diced

1 garlic clove, grated or minced

1 cup (85 g) chopped red Swiss chard stems

2 tablespoons Artisan GF Flour Blend (page 27)

2 pounds (907 g) Yukon gold potatoes, peeled and diced

4 cups (945 ml) GF low-sodium chicken broth or stock

1 cup (240 ml) milk

1 fresh rosemary sprig

½ cup (120 ml) half-and-half, optional

2 teaspoons red wine vinegar

Salt and pepper

1. Cook the bacon in a large saucepan until crispy. Remove with a slotted spoon, keeping the drippings in the pan. When cool, crumble the bacon and set aside.

2. If using fresh corn, boil or steam the ears whole for 5 minutes, then cut the kernels from the cobs when they are cool enough to handle.

3. Add the onion, garlic, and Swiss chard stems to the bacon drippings and sauté over medium heat until soft, about 10 minutes. Add the flour and cook for 1 minute. Add the potatoes, chicken broth, milk, and rosemary. Bring to a boil, turn down to a simmer, and cook for 5 minutes. Remove and discard the rosemary and cook the chowder for another 10 minutes.

4. Add the corn, bring back up to a simmer, and cook for 5 more minutes, until the potatoes and corn are soft. Stir in the half-and-half (if desired) and vinegar, and season with salt and pepper.

5. Using a handheld immersion blender, puree the soup until smooth. Garnish with the reserved bacon and serve.

KIDS CAN . . .

* Collect ingredients from the pantry and refrigerator

* Crumble bacon (once cool)

* Measure ingredients

* Place ingredients in the saucepan

* Use immersion blender (with close supervision)

To make this recipe . . . .

DAIRY/LACTOSE/CASEIN-FREE
- Substitute almond milk (or, for nut allergies, rice or hemp milk) for the cow's milk.
- Omit the half-and-half.

VEGETARIAN
- Omit the bacon, and use 1 to 2 tablespoons olive oil to sauté the onion, garlic, and Swiss chard.
- Substitute GF vegetable broth for the chicken broth.

VEGAN
- Use the dairy-free and vegetarian substitutions.

JUMBO PIGS IN A BLANKET

• MAKES 8 HOT DOGS •

Pigs in a blanket—usually made with small cocktail wieners and croissant dough—are a crowd pleaser. These full-size hot dogs wrapped in gluten-free dough are easier and quicker to prepare, and handy for children to hold and munch on. You can leave them whole to serve as a snack or appetizer, or pair with sides such as French fries to make a full meal. Or you could cut them into pieces, sort of like a sushi roll.

¾ cup (180 ml) warm water (about 115°F/45°C)

1 tablespoon sugar or honey

2¼ teaspoons (1 packet) yeast

3 tablespoons olive oil

1⅓ cups (167 g) Artisan GF Flour Blend (page 27)

1 teaspoon xanthan gum

1 teaspoon salt

8 GF hot dogs (we prefer nitrate-free turkey dogs)

KIDS CAN . . .

* Collect ingredients from the pantry and refrigerator

* Measure ingredients

* Dump ingredients into mixing bowl

* Mix ingredients with a whisk

* Combine wet and dry ingredients and stir

* Cover hot dogs with the dough

1. Combine the water, sugar, and yeast in a bowl and allow to rest for 5 minutes, until the yeast is active and the mixture bubbly with a layer of foam on top. Add 1 tablespoon of the olive oil.

2. In a separate bowl, whisk together the flour, xanthan gum, and salt. Add the yeast mixture and mix to form a dough that is soft and slightly sticky to the touch.

3. Coat your hands with olive oil and divide the dough into 8 equal pieces. Keep a small bowl with 1 tablespoon of the olive oil close for dipping your fingers to help prevent the dough from sticking to your hands. Alternatively, you can add 1 to 2 tablespoons flour to the dough to make it drier, but this will impact the final texture. Wrap one piece of dough around one hot dog and roll between your hands until the entire hot dog is encased in a thin layer of dough. Place on an ungreased baking sheet and repeat with the remaining dough and hot dogs.

4. Brush the wrapped hot dogs with the remaining 1 tablespoon olive oil using a pastry brush. Place the baking sheet in a warm location and allow the dough to rise for 20 minutes.

5. Preheat the oven to 400°F (205°C).

6. Bake the hot dogs for 20 minutes, until the dough is cooked through and golden brown.

To make this recipe . . . .

CORN-FREE

* Use arrowroot flour to make a corn-free version of the Artisan GF Flour Blend (page 26).
* Be wary that some hot dogs contain corn syrup or a similar ingredient.

VEGETARIAN AND VEGAN

* Substitute gluten-free, vegetarian/vegan hot dogs for traditional hot dogs. Be wary that many vegetarian/vegan hot dogs contain vital wheat gluten and are *not* gluten-free.

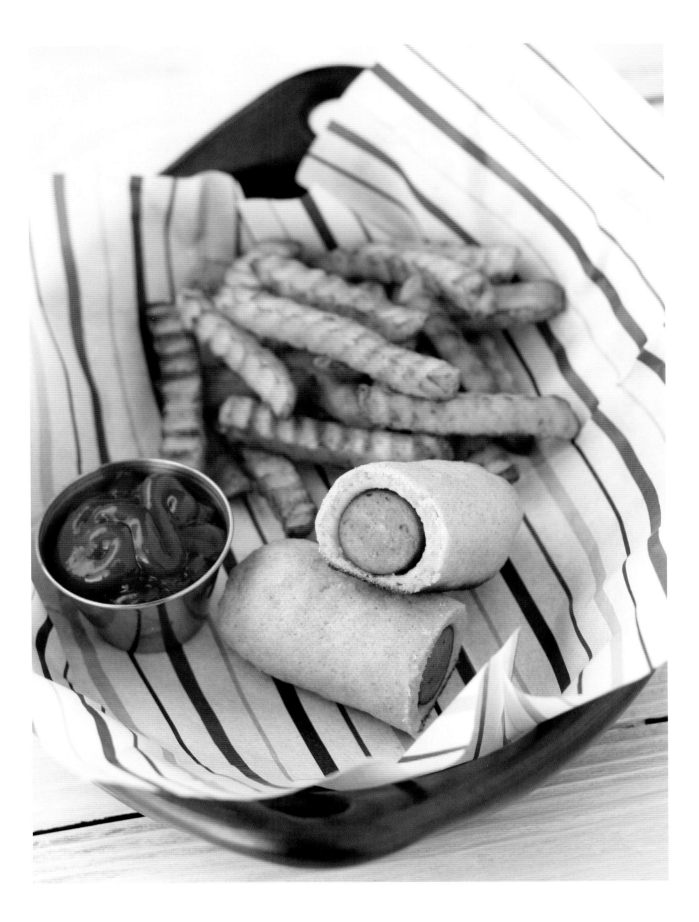

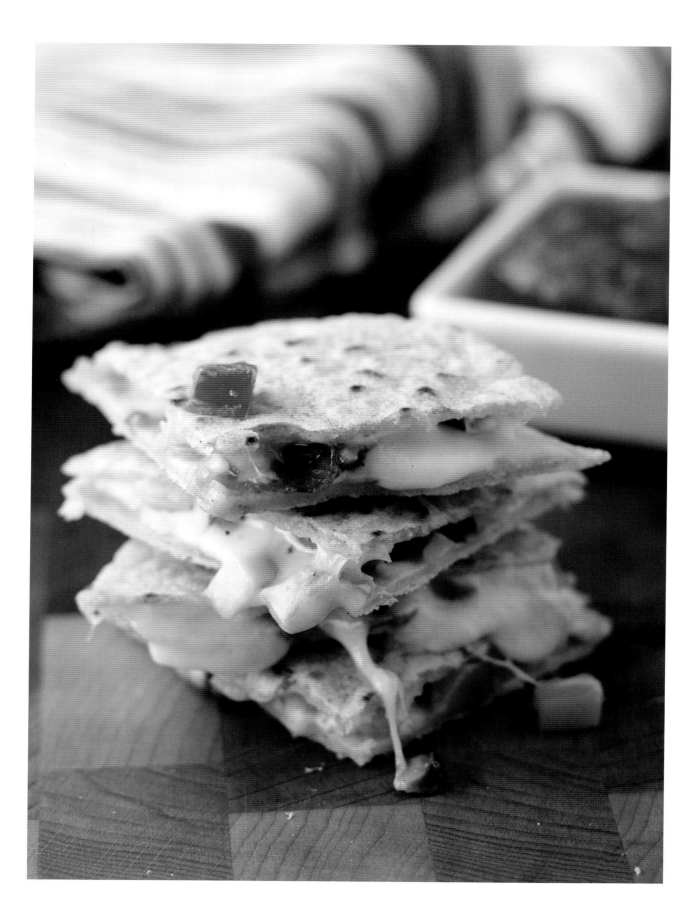

QUESADILLAS

• MAKES 6 QUESADILLAS •

This is a quick and versatile dish that can be made to suit your family's tastes with either plain cheese quesadillas or by adding sautéed vegetables, beans, or shredded chicken, pork, or beef. Or try dipping the quesadillas in Smoky Tomato Salsa (recipe below).

Six 8-inch (20 cm) or twelve 5-inch (13 cm) Tortilla Sandwich Wraps (page 112)

1½ to 3 cups (135 to 270 g) shredded *queso quesadilla*, cheddar, or Monterey Jack cheese

OPTIONAL FILLINGS

Sautéed or grilled vegetables

Black or pinto beans, cooked or canned

Cooked chicken, pork, or beef (grilled, shredded, ground, etc.)

OPTIONAL TOPPINGS

Smoky Tomato Salsa (recipe opposite)

Sour cream

Guacamole

1. Heat a heavy, flat pan over medium-high heat until hot, at least 5 minutes.

2. Place 1 tortilla on a work surface. For a large tortilla, sprinkle half of the tortilla with cheese (about ⅓ to ½ cup) and top with any desired fillings. Fold the naked half of the tortilla over the cheese. For a small tortilla, sprinkle the entire tortilla with cheese (3 to 4 tablespoons), as well as any desired fillings; place a second tortilla on top. Repeat to make the remaining quesadillas.

3. Place 1 quesadilla on the hot pan and cook for about 2 minutes on the first side. Flip and cook for an additional 2 minutes, until the cheese is melted and the surface is toasty. Repeat with the remaining quesadillas.

4. Serve warm with your desired toppings.

Make your own . . .

SMOKY TOMATO SALSA
MAKES ABOUT 4 CUPS

1 jalapeño pepper

½ cup (76 g) corn kernels (omit to make corn-free)

½ medium white onion

3 garlic cloves, peeled

Juice of 1 lime

One 28-ounce (794 g) can diced tomatoes

⅓ to ½ cup (15 to 23 g) cilantro leaves

½ teaspoon ground cumin

½ teaspoon salt

1. Preheat the broiler. Place the pepper on a baking sheet and broil, rotating periodically, until uniformly blackened on all sides. When cool enough to handle, cut off the stem, then de-seed, if you like, for mild salsa; keep in the seeds to make the salsa spicier.

2. Spread the corn kernels out in an even layer on the baking sheet and likewise broil until they begin to char and are roughly equal parts yellow and brown/black.

3. Combine the pepper, corn kernels, and remaining ingredients in a food processor and process until smooth.

KIDS CAN . . .

∗ Collect ingredients from the pantry and refrigerator

∗ Sprinkle cheese on tortillas

To make this recipe . . . .

DAIRY/LACTOSE/CASEIN-FREE AND VEGAN
- Substitute nondairy cheese for the dairy cheese.
- Do not serve with sour cream.

CORN-FREE
- Use arrowroot flour to make a corn-free version of the Artisan GF Flour Blend (page 26) for the tortillas.

PUPUSA POCKETS

• MAKES 8 PUPUSAS •

Salvadoran pupusas are thick corn pancakes traditionally filled with seasoned black beans, pork, and/ or cheese. Our vegetarian version was inspired by our local farmers' market, where a Latin American vendor offered up several varieties for the lunch crowd. They make for a filling meal that really satisfies.

3 cups (360 g) instant corn masa flour (masa harina)

Salt

½ cup (120 ml) olive oil, plus more for cooking

2½ to 3 cups (590 to 710 ml) warm water

One 15-ounce (425 g) can black beans, drained and rinsed

2 tablespoons water

1 tablespoon lime juice

¼ teaspoon ground cumin

¼ teaspoon garlic powder

Pepper

¾ cup (114 g) corn kernels (fresh, frozen, or canned—if using fresh, steam first for 5 minutes)

2½ ounces (68 g) shredded Monterey Jack cheese or *queso quesadilla* (¾ cup)

Olive oil

OPTIONAL TOPPINGS

Smoky Tomato Salsa (page 107)

Sour cream

Guacamole

KIDS CAN . . .

* Collect ingredients from the pantry and refrigerator

* Measure ingredients

* Add ingredients to the mixing bowl and food processor

* Press the food processor buttons

* Mix with a spoon

* Flatten the pupusas after they are shaped in a ball

1. In a large bowl, combine the masa flour and 1 teaspoon salt. Add the olive oil and mix to incorporate. Stir in 2½ cups warm water to make a wet dough. Let rest for 10 minutes.

2. In a food processor, combine the beans, 2 tablespoons water, lime juice, cumin, garlic powder, 1/4 teaspoon salt, and a dash of pepper. Puree until smooth.

3. Cut eight 6-inch (15 cm) squares of parchment paper and set aside.

4. To make the pupusas, divide the dough into 8 equal pieces a little smaller than a tennis ball. Roll 1 piece into a ball and press a hole in the center without going all the way through, making the hole larger until the dough has a large pocket. Add a spoonful each of the black bean filling, corn, and cheese and pinch the edges of the dough together to enclose the filling.

5. Roll the dough between your palms to form a ball, then flatten to about 5 inches (13 cm) in diameter. (If the dough cracks when you try to flatten the first pupusa, add up to ½ cup additional water to the remaining dough, until the dough remains smooth and no longer cracks when you work with it. Combine the divided dough back together, add the water, incorporate, then re-divide.) Repeat to make 8 pupusas, placing each on a square of parchment paper.

6. Heat a skillet over medium heat. Add 1 teaspoon olive oil, then wipe with a piece of paper towel to leave only a thin film of oil. Pick up the pupusas with the parchment paper and flip onto the skillet, in batches. Cook the pupusas for 5 to 8 minutes per side, until cooked through; the crust should be golden brown. Repeat until all of the pupusas are cooked. Serve with salsa, sour cream, and guacamole if desired.

7. Serve fresh and hot, or let cool completely and store in an airtight container in the refrigerator or freezer to reheat later.

To make this recipe . . . .

DAIRY/LACTOSE/CASEIN-FREE AND VEGAN

• Substitute nondairy cheese for the dairy cheese or omit the cheese.

• Do not serve with sour cream.

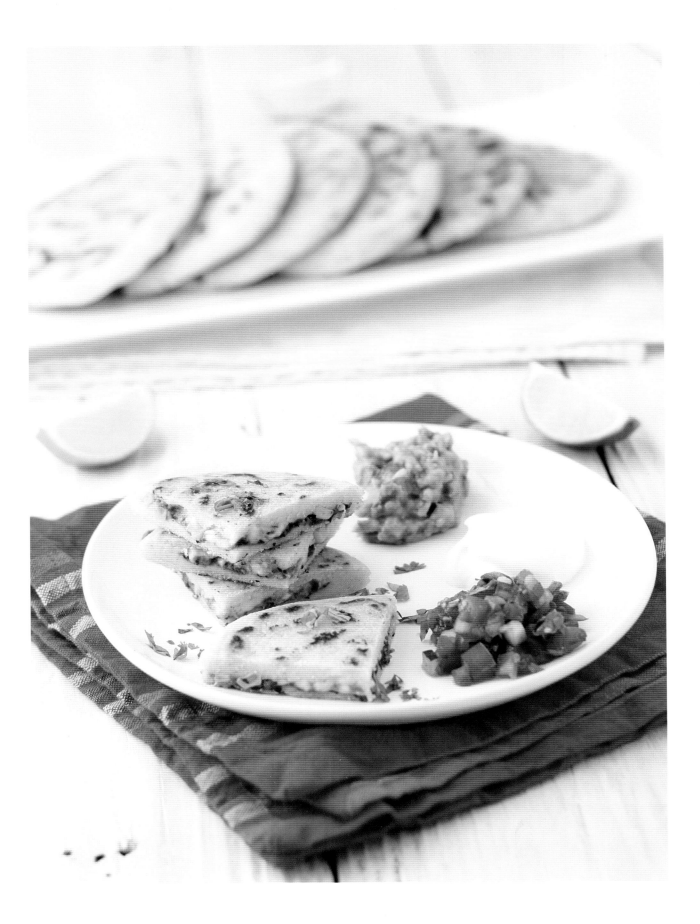

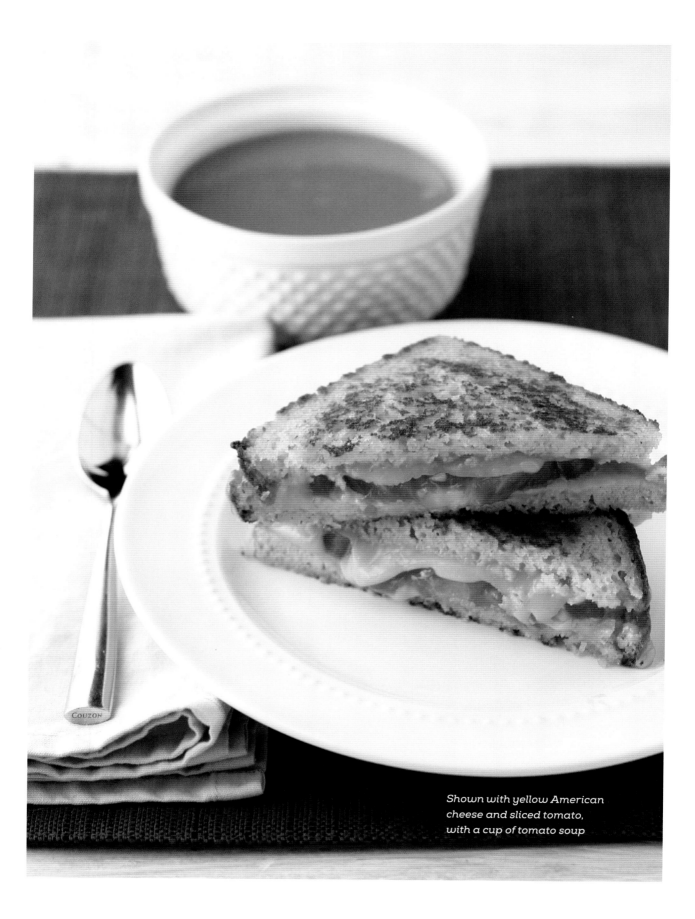

Shown with yellow American cheese and sliced tomato, with a cup of tomato soup

GRILLED CHEESE

• MAKES 2 SANDWICHES •

This American classic—often paired with a cup of tomato soup—can be as simple as cheese and bread or elevated with fillings that make it as appealing to Mom and Dad as it is to the kids. However you choose to build the sandwiches, enjoy them while they are hot and the cheese is gooey.

4 slices Sandwich Bread (page 80)

1 tablespoon butter, room temperature

4 slices American cheese

OPTIONAL FILLINGS

Cooked bacon

Sliced tomato

Sliced salami

Avocado

1. Heat a large skillet over medium-high heat. Spread one side of each piece of bread with butter and place butter-side down in the heated pan. Place 1 piece of cheese on each piece of bread and heat until the cheese is melted and the underside of the bread is golden brown.

2. Place any of the optional fillings on 2 of the slices of bread, then top with another slice of bread, cheese-side down, so that both melted cheeses are in the center. Cut each sandwich in half or quarters and serve.

NOTE: The *refined-sugar-free*, *dairy/lactose/casein-free, egg-free,* and *corn-free* statuses of this recipe are partially dependent on the ingredients in your bread. Our Sandwich Bread (page 80) can be made any combination of the above.

KIDS CAN . . .

✳ Collect ingredients from the pantry and refrigerator

✳ Spread butter on bread

✳ Place cheese on bread

To make this recipe . . . .

DAIRY/LACTOSE/CASEIN-FREE AND VEGAN

• Follow instructions to make a dairy-free version of the Sandwich Bread (page 24).
• Use nondairy cheese.
• Substitute vegan shortening for the butter.

TORTILLA SANDWICH WRAPS

• MAKES SIX 8-INCH (20 CM) OR TWELVE 5-INCH (13 CM) TORTILLAS •

Gluten-free tortillas that are flexible and don't crack or crumble as you're eating them can go a long way toward improving your lunch outlook. Fill them with anything from peanut butter and jelly to ham and cheese, or use them as the base for Quesadillas (page 107) or Cinnamon Chips (page 63). Enjoy them fresh, or freeze for later use.

1½ cups (188 g) Artisan GF Flour Blend (page 27)

1½ teaspoons xanthan gum

1 teaspoon GF baking powder

½ teaspoon salt

3 tablespoons vegan shortening

⅔ cup (160 ml) warm water

1. In a bowl, mix together the flour, xanthan gum, baking powder, and salt. Using your hands or a pastry blender, mix in the shortening until completely incorporated. Add the water and mix with a spoon until a slightly sticky dough forms. Allow the dough to rest for 5 minutes. (After resting, the dough will be soft, but no longer sticky.)

2. Heat a heavy, flat pan over medium-high heat until it is hot, at least 5 minutes.

3. While the pan is heating, divide the dough into 6 equal pieces for large tortillas, or 12 pieces for small tortillas.

4. Roll 1 ball of dough between two pieces of plastic wrap to form an 8-inch (20 cm) or 5-inch (13 cm) tortilla. Remove the top piece of plastic and coat one hand in flour. Lightly dust the flour on the surface of the tortilla, then pick up the entire tortilla using the bottom piece of plastic wrap and set on your flour-coated hand. Remove the bottom piece of plastic wrap and carefully place the tortilla on the hot pan. Cook the tortilla for about 15 seconds on the first side, then use a metal spatula to flip the tortilla and separate from the pan if it sticks. Cook the tortilla for an additional 10 seconds on the second side. Remove the tortilla from the pan and, if desired, wrap in a kitchen towel to keep warm while you make the remaining tortillas.

KIDS CAN . . .

* Collect ingredients from the pantry and refrigerator

* Measure ingredients

* Put ingredients in the mixing bowl

* Mix with hands and spoon

* Help roll out the tortillas

To make this recipe . . . .

CORN-FREE

• Use arrowroot flour to make a corn-free version of the Artisan GF Flour Blend (page 26).

• Check the ingredients of your baking powder, which often contains cornstarch.

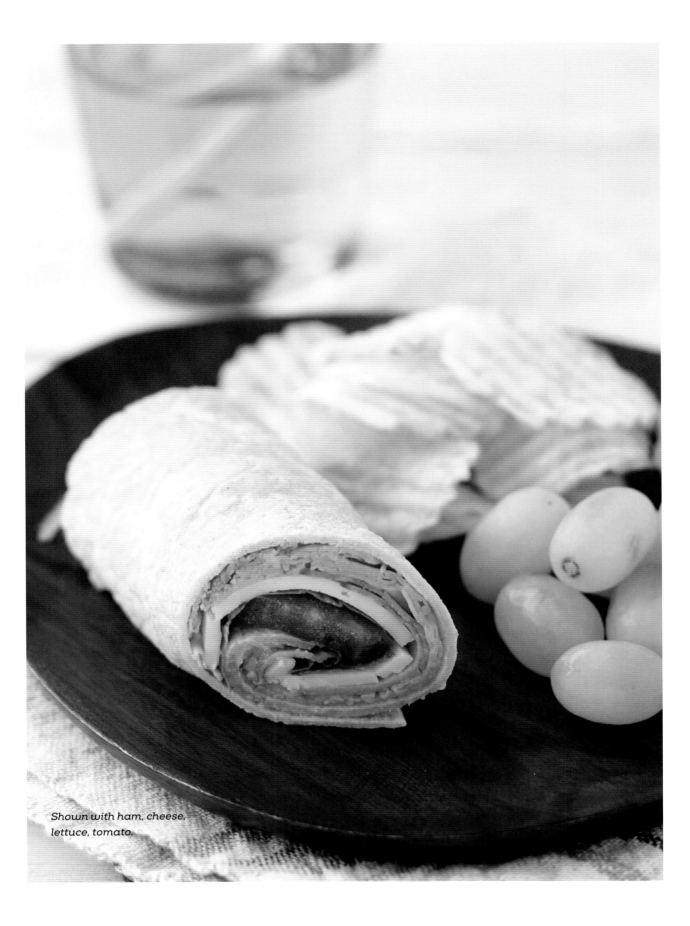

*Shown with ham, cheese,
lettuce, tomato.*

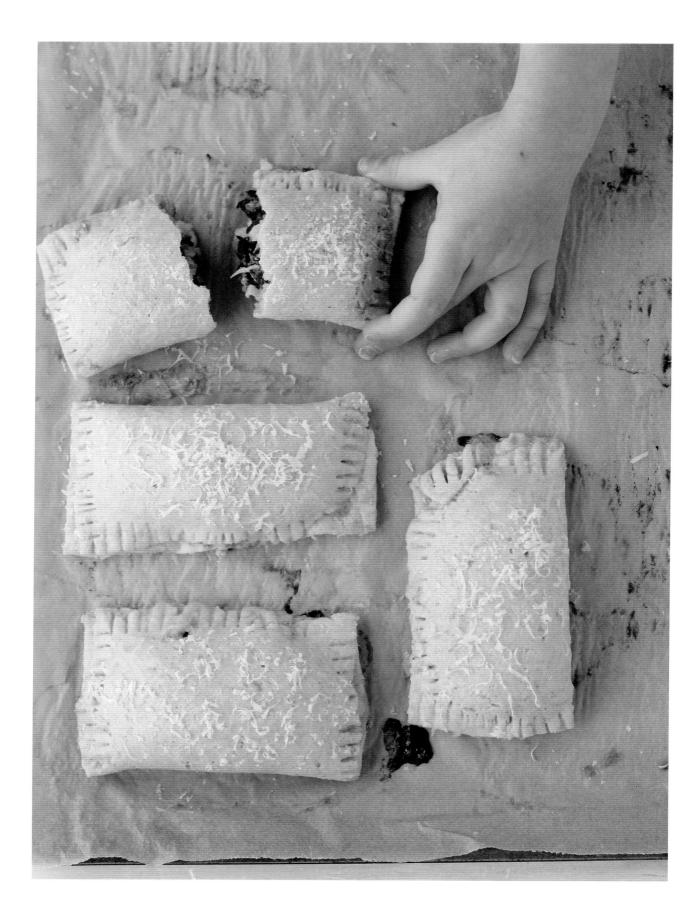

SPANAKOPITA HAND PIES

• MAKES 8 PIES •

Spanakopita is a savory pie filled with spinach and feta and wrapped in layers of glutenous phyllo dough. We have modified the Greek specialty by using an alternative phyllo that we form into individual hand pies. They're sort of like Hot Pockets . . . if Hot Pockets were Greek and filled with spinach.

DOUGH

2 cups plus 2 tablespoons (266 g) Artisan GF Flour Blend (page 27)

1 teaspoon xanthan gum

2 teaspoons GF baking powder

1 teaspoon salt

1 cup (240 ml) seltzer

3 tablespoons olive oil

FILLING

2 tablespoons olive oil

4 scallions, sliced thin

1 small leek with 2 to 3 inches (5 to 8 cm) of green, quartered and sliced thin

8 ounces (227 g) baby spinach

Salt and pepper

1 egg

4 ounces (113 g) feta cheese, crumbled or diced

2 tablespoons grated Parmesan cheese

½ teaspoon ground nutmeg

½ teaspoon ground cumin

TOPPING

1 egg

1 tablespoon grated Parmesan cheese

KIDS CAN . . .

* Collect ingredients from the pantry and refrigerator
* Measure ingredients
* Put ingredients in the mixing bowl
* Mix ingredients with a spoon
* Crack egg
* Crumble feta cheese
* Scoop prepared filling onto rolled-out dough
* Brush pies with egg
* Sprinkle Parmesan cheese

1. Preheat the oven to 375°F (190°C). Line a baking sheet with parchment paper.

2. To make the dough, mix together the flour, xanthan gum, baking powder, and salt in a bowl. Create a well in the center, pour in the seltzer and olive oil, and stir. The dough will be wet. Set aside (the dough will absorb some moisture as it sits).

3. To make the filling, heat the olive oil in a large sauté pan over medium heat. Add the scallions and leek and sauté until very soft, about 5 minutes. Add the spinach and sauté for an additional 5 minutes, until the spinach is wilted and has given off its liquid. Season lightly with salt and pepper, place in a colander, and let drain for

(RECIPE CONTINUES)

To make this recipe . . . .

EGG-FREE
- Omit the egg from the filling.
- Omit the egg wash.

CORN-FREE
- Use arrowroot flour to make a corn-free version of the Artisan GF Flour Blend (page 26).
- Check the ingredients of your baking powder, which often contains cornstarch.

5 minutes. In a large bowl, combine the drained spinach with the egg, feta, Parmesan, nutmeg, and cumin.

4. Roll the dough out between two pieces of plastic wrap to make a rectangle about 10 x 18 inches (25 x 46 cm). Remove the top piece of plastic wrap and cut the dough in half crosswise. Next, cut each rectangle into quarters, creating 8 rectangles each about 5 x 4½ inches (13 x 12 cm).

5. Place a scant ¼ cup (60 ml) filling on one half of a rectangle, leaving a ½-inch (1 cm) border on three sides. Use the plastic wrap under the dough (or flour-dusted fingertips) to lift up the half without the filling and fold it over the filling. Pull the plastic wrap off and use a fork to press the edges of the pies together. Repeat with the remaining dough and filling to make 8 pies.

6. Dust your hands with flour to prevent the pies from sticking to your hands and carefully move the pies off the plastic wrap to the prepared baking sheet.

7. To top the pies, beat the remaining egg in a small bowl and use a pastry brush to coat the tops with egg. Sprinkle with Parmesan cheese. Bake for 25 minutes, until golden brown on top.

8. Serve fresh and hot or, once completely cool, store in an airtight container in the refrigerator or freezer and reheat later in a 350°F (175°C) oven or the microwave (times vary based on microwave strength; watch carefully).

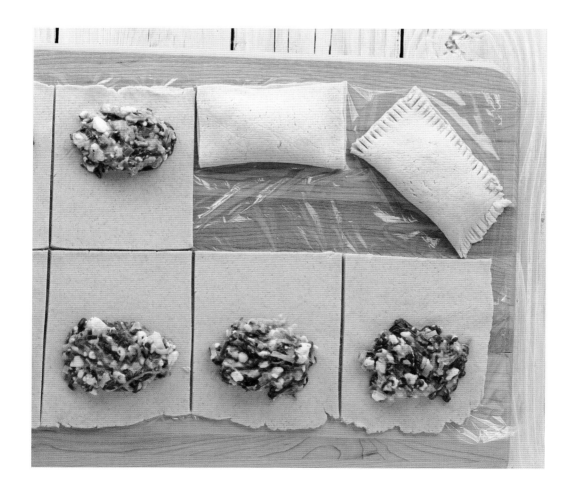

FISH STICKS

This homemade take on a freezer-section convenience food starts with a beautiful fillet of fresh fish. The sticks are surprisingly easy to make and, like our Chicken Fingers (page 128), they're baked instead of fried. Pair them with our tangy tartar sauce that has just enough zip for parents but not too much for the kiddos.

FISH STICKS

1 pound (454 g) haddock, cod, or pollock

1 cup (118 g) GF bread crumbs (see page 75 to make your own)

¼ cup (23 g) grated Parmesan cheese, optional

¼ teaspoon dried oregano

¼ teaspoon dried basil

¼ teaspoon garlic powder

Salt and pepper

1 egg

1 tablespoon water

¼ cup (31 g) Artisan GF Flour Blend (page 27)

Olive oil

TARTAR SAUCE

½ cup (110 g) mayonnaise

¼ cup (47 g) diced dill pickle

1½ tablespoons minced onion

1 tablespoon lemon juice

1 tablespoon capers, chopped

1 tablespoon Dijon mustard

5 shakes GF hot sauce

Salt and pepper

1. Preheat the oven to 400°F (205°C). Place a wire rack on a baking pan and spray the rack with nonstick cooking spray or olive oil from a mister.

2. Rinse the fish and pat dry. Cut into 1½ x 4-inch (4 x 10 cm) strips.*

3. In a shallow bowl, combine the bread crumbs, Parmesan (if using), oregano, basil, garlic powder, ¼ teaspoon salt (omit if using Parmesan), and ¼ teaspoon pepper. In a second bowl, make an egg wash by whisking together the egg and water.** In a third bowl, mix the flour with a little salt and pepper.

4. Place the bowls in a row with the flour first, followed by the egg wash, and then the bread crumb mixture. Dip a piece of fish in the flour, shaking off any excess, then coat with egg wash. Finally, coat with bread crumbs and place on the prepared wire rack. (For the best results, use one hand for the flour and bread crumbs and the other hand for the egg.) Repeat with the remaining pieces of fish.

5. Using an olive oil mister, coat the tops of each piece of fish with a light misting of olive oil, just enough to moisten, but not saturate, the bread crumbs. Bake the fish sticks for 15 to 20 minutes, until golden brown and cooked through.

6. To make the tartar sauce, combine all of the ingredients in a bowl, mix to combine, and chill before serving, if desired. The sauce will keep for up to 3 days in the refrigerator.

7. Serve the fish sticks with the tartar sauce.

*It's more important to have fish sticks of even thickness for uniform cooking than to exactly match our recommended size; work with the cut of fish you have.

**If you don't have an olive oil mister, adjust the breading procedure by following the egg-free instructions.

(RECIPE CONTINUES)

* Collect ingredients from the pantry and refrigerator

* Measure dry ingredients

* Dump dry ingredients into bowls

* Mix dry ingredients with a whisk, spoon, or fork

* Crack the egg and make the egg wash

* Bread the fish sticks

* Mist the fish sticks with olive oil

NOTE: The *refined-sugar-free*, *dairy/lactose/casein-free*, *egg-free*, and *corn-free* statuses of this recipe are partially dependent on the ingredients in your bread crumbs. Our Sandwich Bread (page 80) can be made any combination of the above.

To make this recipe . . . .

DAIRY/LACTOSE/CASEIN-FREE AND REFINED-SUGAR-FREE

* Check the ingredients of your bread crumbs.

EGG-FREE

* Make sure you're using egg-free bread crumbs.
* Omit the flour and replace the egg wash with 3 tablespoons olive oil.
* Dip each fish stick in the olive oil, then coat with bread crumbs and transfer to the wire rack.

CORN-FREE

* Check the ingredients of your bread crumbs.
* Use arrowroot flour to make a corn-free version of the Artisan GF Flour Blend (page 26).

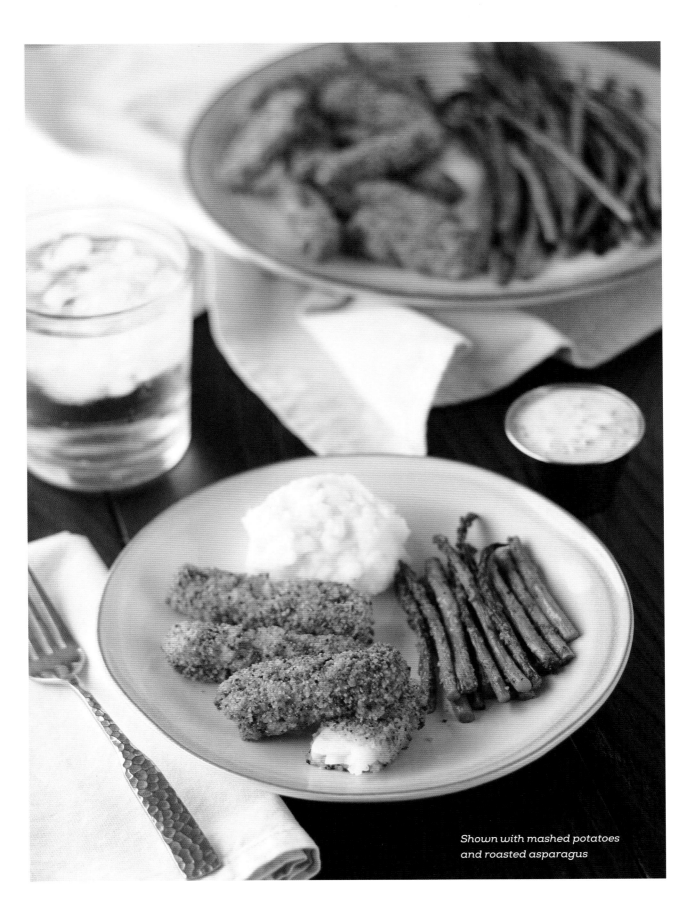

*Shown with mashed potatoes
and roasted asparagus*

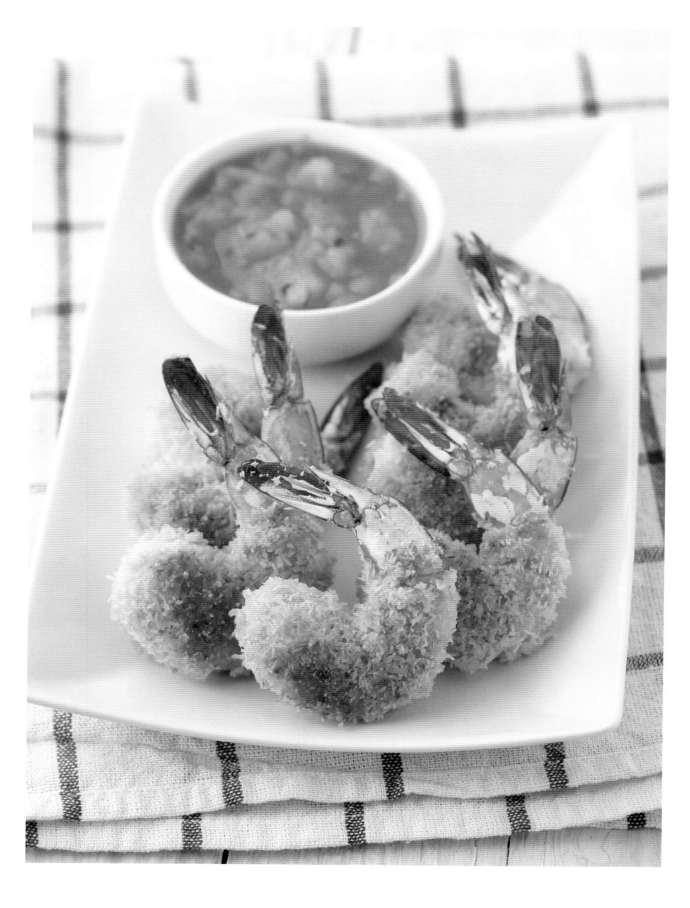

COCONUT SHRIMP
WITH MANGO DIPPING SAUCE

• MAKES 30 TO 40 SHRIMP •

A bright, slightly sweet mango dipping sauce is the perfect counterpoint to double-crusted coconut shrimp.

MANGO DIPPING SAUCE

1 mango, diced small

Zest of ½ navel orange, cut into very thin strips

Juice of 1 navel orange

6 tablespoons (128 g) honey

2 teaspoons grated fresh ginger (¾-inch/2 cm piece)

2 garlic cloves, grated or minced

½ teaspoon chili sauce

COCONUT SHRIMP

1½ cups (57 g) GF crisp rice cereal

1½ cups (122 g) unsweetened dehydrated shredded coconut

¾ teaspoon salt

1 egg

½ cup (120 ml) olive oil

2 pounds (907 g) peeled and deveined jumbo shrimp (16/20 count), tails on

KIDS CAN . . .

* Collect ingredients from the pantry and refrigerator

* Measure ingredients for the sauce

* Juice the orange using a citrus reamer over a strainer to catch the seeds

* Put the ingredients in the saucepan

* Press the food processor buttons

* Measure and mix together the dry ingredients

* Crack the egg

* Dip the shrimp

1. To make the dipping sauce, combine the mango, orange zest, and orange juice in a small saucepan and bring to a boil. Reduce the heat and simmer for 10 minutes, until the mixture is reduced by about half. Add the honey, ginger, garlic, and chili sauce and cook for an additional 2 minutes. If desired, puree to make a smoother sauce. Chill in the refrigerator until serving.

2. Preheat the oven to 400°F (205°C). Place a wire rack on a baking pan and spray the rack with nonstick cooking spray or olive oil from a mister.

3. To prepare the shrimp, pulse the cereal in the food processor until very fine. In a shallow bowl, combine the ground-up cereal, coconut, and salt. In a separate bowl, whisk the egg. Place the olive oil in a third bowl.

4. Rinse the shrimp and pat dry. Dip one shrimp in the beaten egg, holding it up to let excess egg drip off. Next dip the shrimp in the coconut mixture, then in the olive oil, and finally back in the coconut mixture a second time. Place on the prepared wire rack. Repeat to coat the remaining shrimp.

5. Bake the shrimp for 12 minutes, until cooked through.* Switch the oven to broil and broil until golden, 1 to 2 minutes. Flip the shrimp and broil the other side until golden brown. Serve hot with the dipping sauce.

*If using smaller shrimp (higher count per pound), decrease the bake time since they'll cook through faster than 16/20 count shrimp.

To make this recipe . . . .

TREE-NUT-FREE

• Whether you need to do anything to make this recipe tree-nut-free depends on your perspective on coconuts. The US FDA classifies coconut as a tree nut, which would make it a Top 8 allergen. Meanwhile, Food Allergy Research & Education (formerly the Food Allergy and Anaphylaxis Network) and a number of peer-reviewed studies conclude just the opposite.[31]

REFINED-SUGAR-FREE

• Check the ingredients of your gluten-free crisp rice cereal—some contain sugar, while others are sweetened with an alternative sweetener such as brown rice syrup.

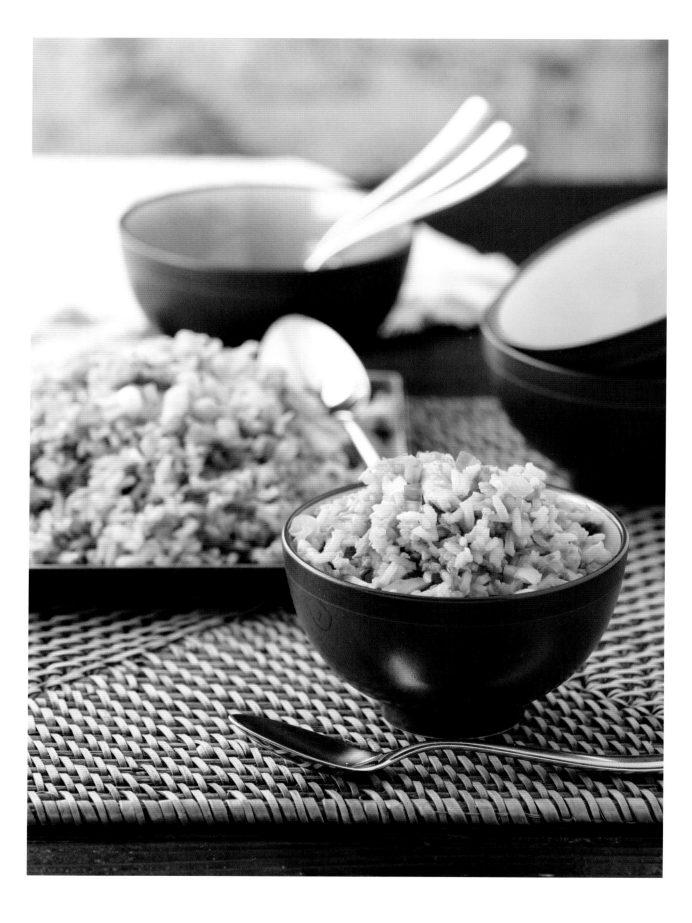

CHICKEN FRIED RICE

• MAKES 4 TO 6 SERVINGS •

What can be better than a quick, easy, one-skillet (or wok) dinner? Fried rice is all of those things and is inherently flexible. Feel free to substitute different or more vegetables to meet your family's taste preferences. This meal is a great way to use up leftovers.

4 tablespoons olive oil

1 tablespoon grated fresh ginger (1- to 2-inch/2.5 to 5 cm piece)

2 garlic cloves, grated or minced

1 chicken breast, cut into small, thin strips

1 large carrot, finely shredded

2 eggs

3 cups (500 g) cooled cooked rice (from 1 cup uncooked)

¼ cup (60 ml) GF tamari wheat-free low-sodium soy sauce or GF soy sauce

1 teaspoon sesame oil

5 scallions, chopped

KIDS CAN . . .

* Collect ingredients from the pantry and refrigerator

* Measure the tamari

* Crack eggs into a bowl

1. Heat 2 tablespoons of the olive oil in a wok or large sauté pan over medium-high heat. Add the ginger and garlic and cook until fragrant, about 30 seconds. Add the chicken and cook for 1 minute. Add the shredded carrot and cook until the chicken is done and the carrots are soft, 3 to 5 minutes.

2. Move the chicken and carrots to the perimeter. Add the eggs to the center, and scramble until nearly done. Move the eggs to the perimeter.

3. Add the remaining 2 tablespoons olive oil to the center and heat for a few seconds. Add the rice and stir-fry for a few minutes, until warm and any clumps have broken up. Add the tamari, sesame oil, and scallions. Toss all the ingredients together and stir-fry for an additional minute, until the flavors have melded.

Make your own . . .

SOY-FREE "SOY" SAUCE: In a medium saucepan, combine 1½ cups (355 ml) water, ¼ cup (60 ml) GF beef broth, 4 teaspoons balsamic vinegar, 2 teaspoons molasses, and a pinch each of ground ginger, pepper, and garlic powder. Reduce over medium-high heat to 1 cup (240 ml). Store refrigerated for up to 1 week.

To make this recipe . . . .

SOY-FREE
* Substitute coconut aminos for the soy sauce, or make your own soy-free "soy" sauce (see above).

EGG-FREE
* Omit the eggs.

VEGETARIAN
* Substitute extra firm tofu for the chicken, patted dry and diced.

VEGAN
* Use the egg-free and vegetarian substitutions.

CHICKEN AND BROCCOLI ASIAN NOODLE BOWL

• MAKES 4 SERVINGS •

Our kids love noodle bowls. This one combines our favorite flavors with notes of sweet, salty, sour, and a touch of spice (which can be increased, and often is by the parents in our home).

2 chicken breasts

4 tablespoons GF tamari wheat-free low-sodium soy sauce or GF soy sauce

1 broccoli crown (head)

2 cups (475 ml) water

¼ cup (60 ml) rice vinegar

2 tablespoons fish sauce

2 tablespoons packed brown sugar

2 tablespoons cornstarch

1 teaspoon chili garlic sauce

1 teaspoon garlic powder

1 tablespoon olive oil

10 ounces (283 g) thin rice noodles

KIDS CAN . . .

* Collect ingredients from the pantry and refrigerator

* Measure ingredients

* Dump sauce ingredients in the mixing bowl

* Mix ingredients together with a whisk

1. Bring a large pot of water to a boil.

2. Slice the chicken breasts in half lengthwise to make a total of 4 thin breasts. Thinly slice the thin breasts to make strips. Combine the chicken strips with 1 tablespoon of the soy sauce in a bowl and set aside. Cut the broccoli into individual florets. Halve or quarter the florets as necessary so they're all roughly equal in size. Set aside.

3. Mix together the remaining 3 tablespoons soy sauce, 1 cup of the water, the rice vinegar, fish sauce, sugar, cornstarch, chili garlic sauce, and garlic powder. Set aside.

4. Heat a large skillet over medium-high heat. Add the broccoli and remaining 1 cup of water to the pan and cover. Steam the broccoli for 3 minutes, until slightly tender and still very green. Remove the broccoli from the skillet and drain any extra water.

5. Wipe the large skillet dry and heat over medium-high heat. Add the olive oil. Add the chicken and sauté for 3 to 4 minutes, until cooked through, being conscious not to stir too much, allowing the chicken to brown and develop great flavor. Remove the chicken and set aside.

6. Meanwhile, when the water in the pot comes to a boil, add the rice noodles and boil until just shy of al dente, about 3 minutes. Drain.

7. Add the soy sauce mixture to the skillet and bring to a boil, cooking until it turns clear and begins to thicken, about 2 minutes. Return the chicken and broccoli to the pan, remove from the heat, and add the noodles. Toss to coat everything with the sauce.

To make this recipe . . . .

SOY-FREE
* Substitute coconut aminos for the soy sauce, or make your own soy-free "soy" sauce (page 123).

FISH-FREE
* Omit the fish sauce.

CORN-FREE
* Substitute another thickener for the cornstarch, such as tapioca starch, potato starch, or arrowroot flour.

REFINED-SUGAR-FREE
* Substitute honey for the brown sugar.
* Check the ingredients of your fish sauce, which can contain sugar.

VEGETARIAN AND VEGAN
* Omit the fish sauce.
* Substitute extra firm tofu, patted dry and diced, for the chicken.

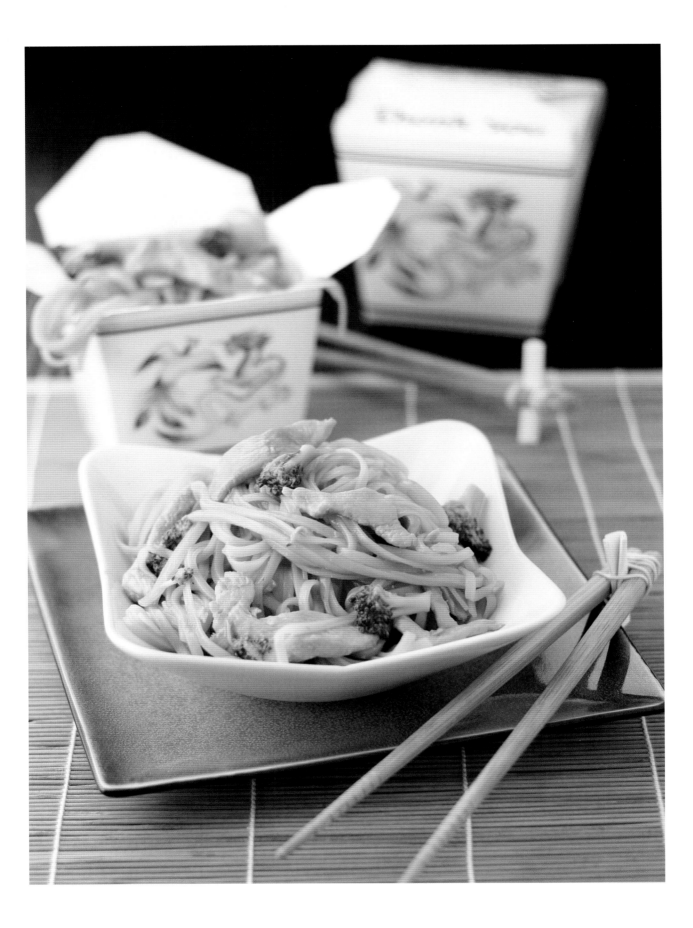

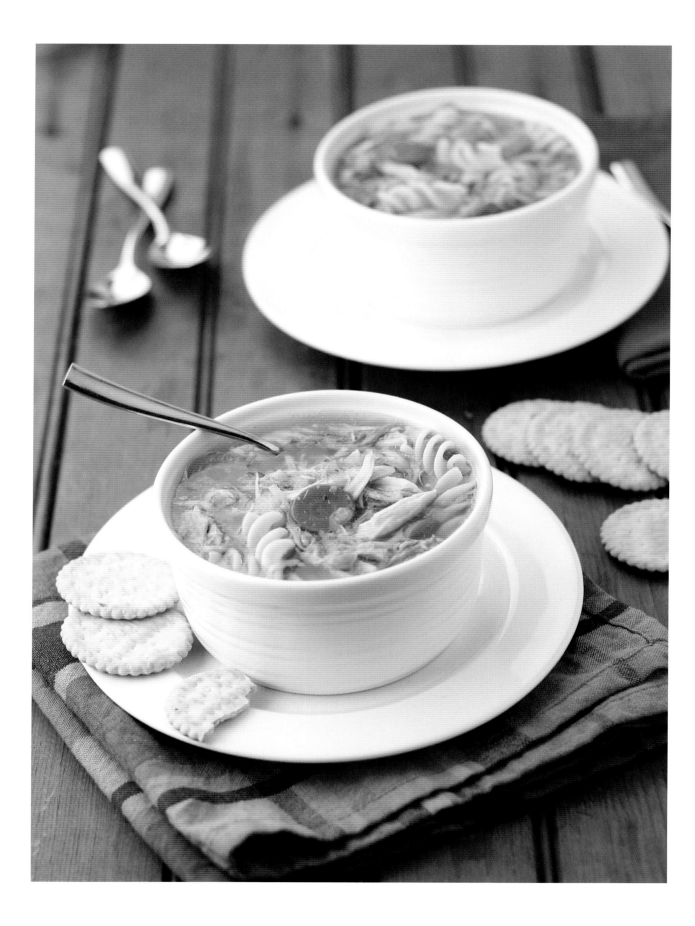

SLOW COOKER CHICKEN NOODLE SOUP

• MAKES 6 SERVINGS •

When the temperature dips and the snow starts to fly, there's nothing like coming in from the cold to a hot bowl of soul-warming chicken noodle soup. Fortified with the flavors of a whole chicken, ours is a rich and satisfying meal—and the slow cooker does most of the work for you.

2 celery stalks, diced (about ¾ cup/100 g)

2 small carrots, sliced into "coins" (about ¾ cup/100 g)

1 medium onion, diced (about ¾ cup/105 g)

2 bay leaves

1 teaspoon dried thyme

½ teaspoon salt

½ teaspoon pepper

1 whole chicken, quartered

2 cups (475 ml) GF low-sodium chicken broth or stock

2 cups (475 ml) water

1 cup (100 g) GF short pasta (e.g., macaroni shells)

KIDS CAN . . .

* Collect ingredients from the pantry and refrigerator

* Measure ingredients

* Count bay leaves

* Place ingredients in slow cooker

1. Combine the celery, carrot, onion, bay leaves, thyme, salt, and pepper in the slow cooker. Place the chicken quarters on top of the vegetables and pour the broth and water over the top to fully submerge the ingredients. Cover and cook on high for 5 hours, until the chicken is cooked through and shreds easily.

2. Remove the chicken pieces from the soup and set aside to cool. Meanwhile, add the pasta to the soup, cover, and cook on high for 30 minutes more, until the pasta is tender.

3. When the chicken is cool enough to handle, remove the skin and discard. Remove the 2 breasts and reserve for another use, such as chicken salad. Shred the remaining meat (thighs, legs, etc.), discarding any fat and bones.

4. Add the shredded meat to the simmering soup. Discard the bay leaves and, if desired, skim off any fat before serving the soup.

NOTE: If you have a large slow cooker and want to feed a crowd, you can double all the quantities (except the whole chicken). Include the two reserved chicken breasts in the soup.

To make this recipe . . . .

CORN-FREE

• Make sure you use a corn-free gluten-free pasta, such as those made from brown rice or quinoa.

CHICKEN FINGERS

• MAKES 8 CHICKEN FINGERS •

Chicken fingers are great kid-friendly finger food. By oven roasting rather than pan- or deep-frying, we improve the nutrition but sacrifice none of the flavor. While many kids might opt to dip in ketchup, our girls prefer a homemade honey mustard, made with equal parts honey and Dijon mustard.

1 pound (454 g) chicken tenderloins (whole); or 2 boneless, skinless breasts, cut into 4 strips each

1 cup (118 g) GF bread crumbs (see page 75 to make your own)

¼ teaspoon dried oregano

¼ teaspoon dried basil

¼ teaspoon garlic powder

Salt and pepper

1 egg

1 tablespoon water

¼ cup (31 g) Artisan GF Flour Blend (page 27)

Olive oil

1. Preheat the oven to 400°F (205°C). Place a wire rack on a baking pan and spray the rack with nonstick cooking spray or olive oil from a mister.

2. If you are using chicken tenderloins, remove the tendons: Place the tenderloin with the tendon-side down on a cutting board. Place the back of your knife (not the sharp blade side as that will cut the tendon) on top of the tendon and hold the tendon to the board with your finger. Use your knife to slide the chicken off the tendon with firm pressure, pushing away from your finger holding the tendon. If the tendon breaks that's fine; you mostly want to remove the large, tough part that sticks out of the meat.

3. In a shallow bowl, combine the bread crumbs, oregano, basil, garlic powder, ¼ teaspoon salt, and ¼ teaspoon pepper. In a second bowl, make an egg wash by whisking together the egg and water.* In a third bowl, mix the flour with a little salt and pepper.

4. Place the bowls in a row with the flour first, then the egg wash, and then the bread crumb mixture. Dip a piece of chicken in flour, shaking off any excess, then coat with egg wash. Finally, coat with bread crumbs and place on the prepared wire rack. (For the best results, use one hand for the flour and bread crumbs and the other hand for the egg.) Repeat to coat the remaining pieces of chicken.

5. Using an olive oil mister, coat the tops of each piece of chicken lightly with olive oil, just enough to moisten, but not saturate, the bread crumbs. Bake for 20 minutes, until golden brown and cooked through.

*If you don't have an olive oil mister, adjust the breading procedure by following the egg-free instructions below.

NOTE: The *refined-sugar-free*, *dairy/lactose/casein-free*, *egg-free*, and *corn-free* statuses of this recipe are partially dependent on the ingredients in your bread crumbs. Our Sandwich Bread (page 80) can be made any combination of the above.

KIDS CAN . . .

* Collect ingredients from the pantry and refrigerator

* Measure dry ingredients

* Dump dry ingredients into their bowls

* Mix dry ingredients with a whisk, spoon, or fork

* Crack the egg and make the egg wash

* Bread the chicken fingers

* Mist the chicken fingers with olive oil

To make this recipe . . . .

EGG-FREE
- Omit the flour and replace the egg wash with 3 tablespoons olive oil.
- Make sure you're using egg-free bread crumbs.

- Dip each chicken tender in the olive oil, then coat with bread crumbs and transfer to the wire rack.

CORN-FREE
- Check the ingredients of your bread crumbs.
- Use arrowroot flour to make a corn-free version of the Artisan GF Flour Blend (page 26).

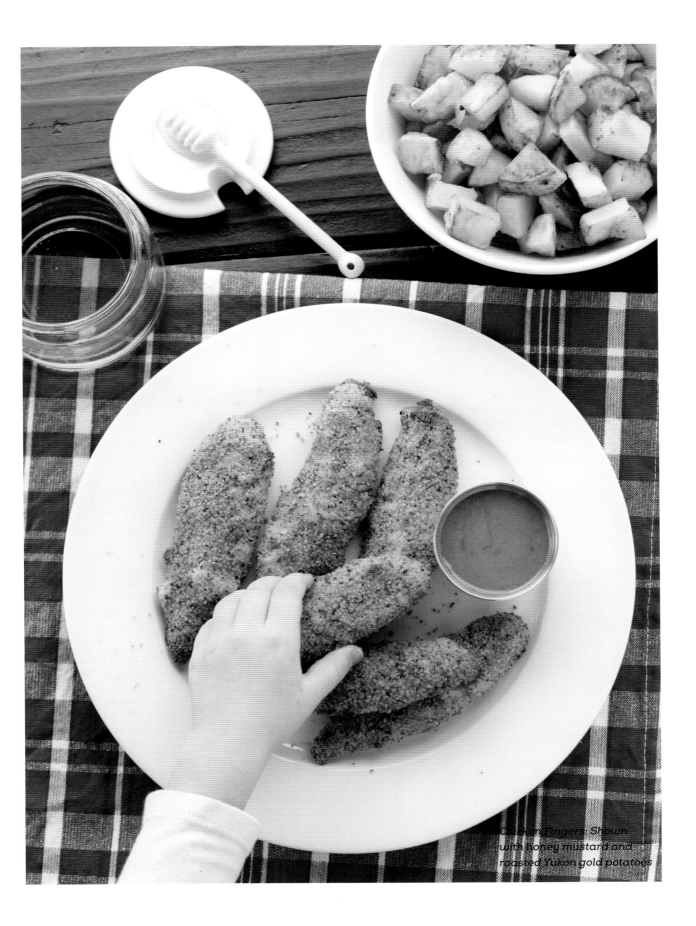

Chicken Fingers: Shown with honey mustard and roasted Yukon gold potatoes

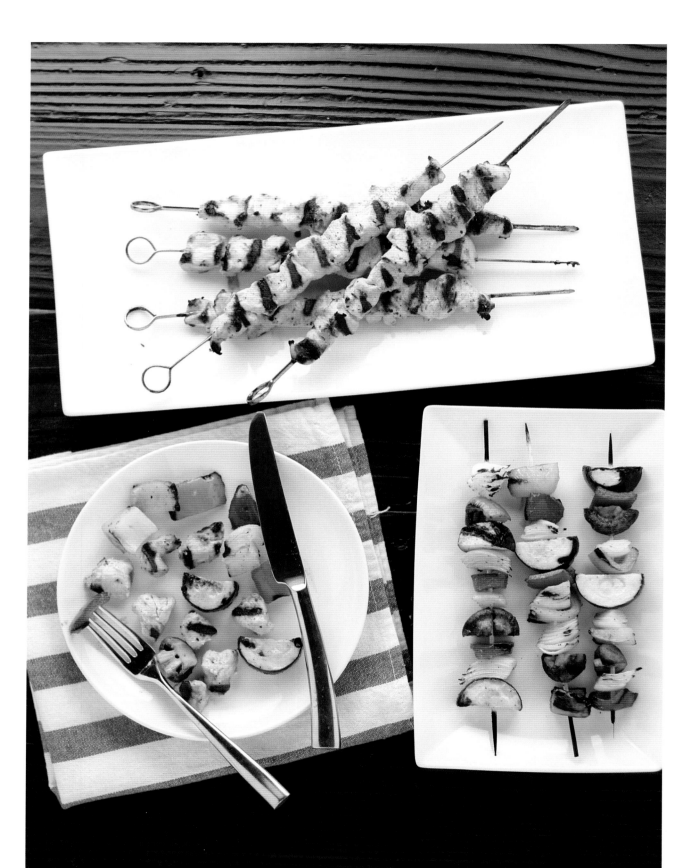

MEDITERRANEAN CHICKEN SKEWERS

• MAKES 4 TO 6 SERVINGS •

These chicken skewers are easy to make, flavorful, and moist. The yogurt in the marinade serves two purposes: It is a natural tenderizer and also adds deeper flavors to the tender chicken. Try pairing the chicken skewers with grilled vegetables, such as peppers, onions, and mushrooms, as we did in the photographed version.

MARINADE

¼ cup (60 g) plain yogurt

Juice of ½ lemon (about 2 tablespoons)

2 tablespoons olive oil

1 tablespoon white wine vinegar

1 garlic clove, grated or minced

¼ teaspoon dried oregano

¼ teaspoon paprika

¼ teaspoon pepper

Pinch of salt (about ⅛ teaspoon)

1¼ pounds (567 g) boneless, skinless chicken breasts or thighs, cut into cubes

1. Combine all of the marinade ingredients in a large bowl. Add the chicken and toss to coat. Cover the bowl and marinate in the refrigerator for at least 3 hours or up to 24.

2. Preheat a grill.

3. Skewer the chicken cubes onto bamboo or metal skewers.* Grill over medium-high heat, turning, until the chicken is cooked through, about 10 minutes.

* If using bamboo skewers, soak them in water for 15 minutes before using.

KIDS CAN . . .

* Collect ingredients from the pantry and refrigerator

* Measure the ingredients

* Place the ingredients in the mixing bowl

* Mix ingredients with a spoon

To make this recipe . . . .

DAIRY/LACTOSE/CASEIN-FREE
• Use nondairy yogurt.

VEGETARIAN
• Substitute extra firm tofu, patted dry and cubed, for the chicken.

VEGAN
• Use the dairy-free and vegetarian substitutions.

TERIYAKI CHICKEN

• MAKES 4 SERVINGS •

Teriyaki, a traditional Japanese dish, has a sweet and slightly salty flavor that kids love. The chicken has a beautiful sheen and the combination of soy, mirin, sesame, and ginger forms the flavor foundation. Serve with rice.

1 tablespoon olive oil

6 boneless chicken thighs (1¼ pounds/567 g), trimmed of fat

¼ cup (60 ml) sake

¼ cup (60 ml) water

3 tablespoons GF tamari wheat-free low-sodium soy sauce or GF soy sauce

3 tablespoons mirin*

2 tablespoons packed brown sugar

2 teaspoons grated fresh ginger (¾-inch/2 cm piece)

1 teaspoon sesame oil

2 garlic cloves, grated or minced

1 bunch scallions, green part only, cut into 3-inch (8 cm) sections

1. Heat the olive oil in a sauté pan over medium-high heat. Add the chicken and cook for about 5 minutes per side, until cooked through, being conscious not to move the chicken too much, allowing it to brown and develop great flavor.

2. While the chicken is cooking, in a small bowl, combine the sake, water, soy sauce, mirin, sugar, ginger, sesame oil, and garlic.

3. Remove the chicken from the pan. Add the sauce to the pan, turn down the heat to low, and simmer for 2 minutes. Return the chicken to the pan with the scallions and simmer, turning the chicken once to coat in the sauce, for an additional 5 minutes.

*If you cannot find mirin, substitute rice vinegar and increase the brown sugar to 3 tablespoons.

KIDS CAN . . .

* Collect ingredients from the pantry and refrigerator

* Measure the ingredients

* Place the ingredients in a bowl

* Mix with a whisk, spoon, or fork

To make this recipe . . . .

SOY-FREE
- Substitute coconut aminos for the soy sauce, or make your own soy-free "soy" sauce (page 123).

VEGETARIAN AND VEGAN
- Substitute extra firm tofu, patted dry and diced, for the chicken.

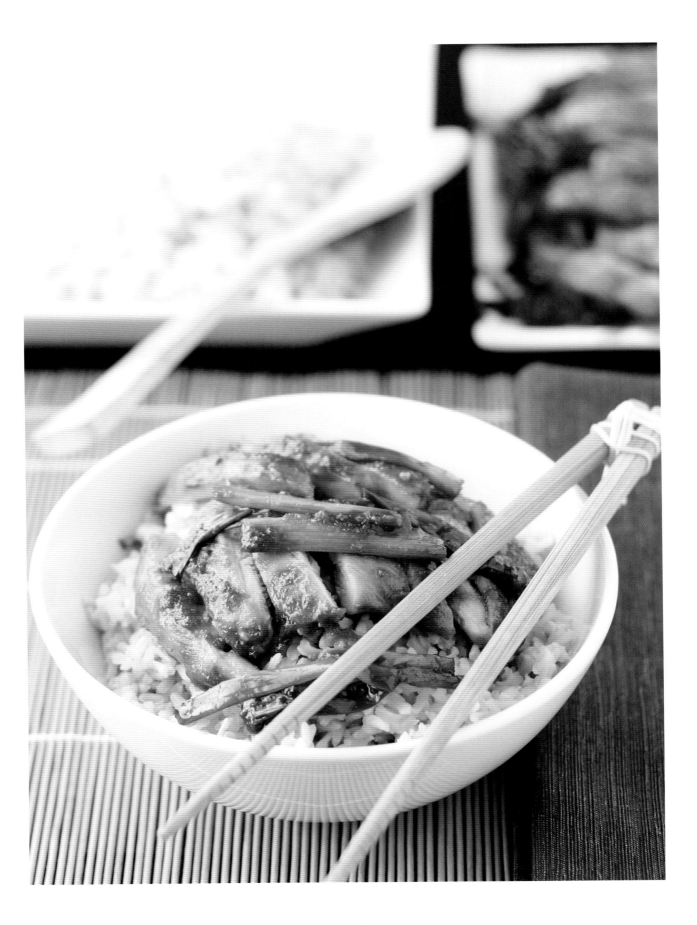

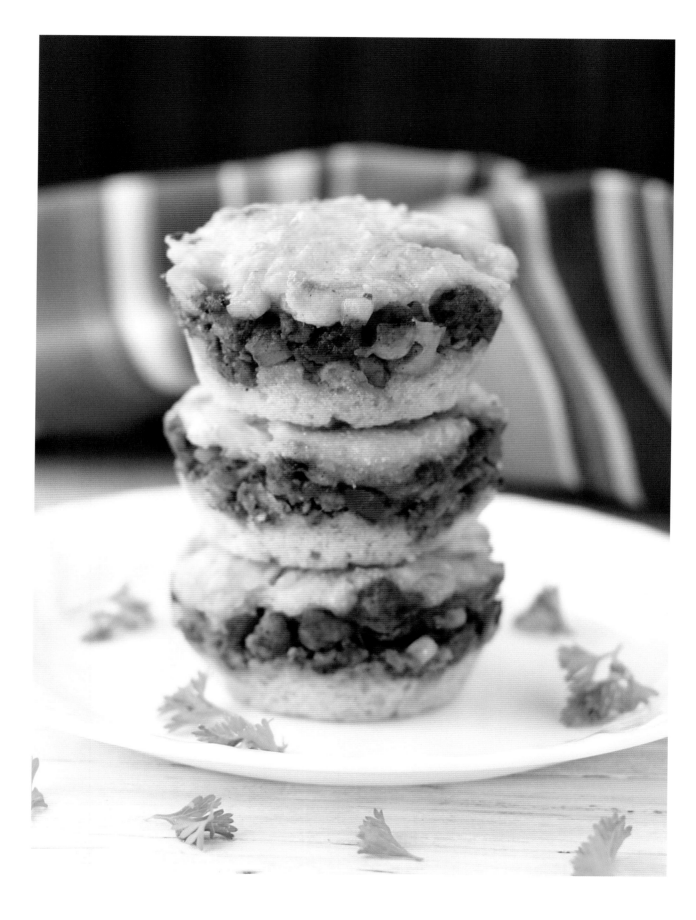

CORNBREAD TACO MUFFINS

• MAKES 20 MUFFINS •

This new twist on an old favorite turns cornbread into a more versatile meal. You can make them ahead of time, freeze, and reheat as needed. They also travel well as a portable lunch or dinner.

FILLING

1 tablespoon olive oil

½ red bell pepper, diced

½ medium yellow onion, diced

1 pound (454 g) ground turkey (93% lean)

1 tablespoon ground cumin

1 tablespoon chili powder

1 teaspoon dried oregano

1 teaspoon garlic powder

½ cup (76 g) corn kernels (fresh, frozen, or canned—if using fresh, steam first for 5 minutes)

1½ cups (411 g) diced tomatoes or one 14.5-ounce (411 g) can no-salt-added diced tomatoes

Salt and pepper

CORNBREAD

1 cup (125 g) Artisan GF Flour Blend (page 27)

1 cup (170 g) cornmeal

1 tablespoon GF baking powder

1 teaspoon salt

1 cup (240 ml) milk

2 eggs

1 tablespoon honey

¼ cup (½ stick, 56 g) butter, melted

½ cup (76 g) corn kernels (fresh, frozen, or canned—if using fresh, steam first for 5 minutes)

1 cup (80 to 90 g) shredded sharp cheddar cheese or *queso quesadilla*

1. To make the filling, heat the olive oil in a large sauté pan over medium-high heat. Add the red pepper and onion and sauté until softened, 3 to 4 minutes. Add the ground turkey and sauté until brown and cooked through. Add the cumin, chili powder, oregano, and garlic powder and stir to combine. Stir in the corn and tomatoes and sauté for about 1 minute. Season with salt and pepper to taste, remove from the heat, and set aside.

2. Preheat the oven to 375°F (190°C). Grease 20 cups of two 12-cup muffin tins with butter or nonstick cooking spray.

3. To make the cornbread, mix together the flour, cornmeal, baking powder, and salt. Add the milk, eggs, and honey and whisk to combine. Stir in the melted butter, then stir in the corn and cheese. (See the variation, below, for instructions for using the batter to make traditional cornbread.)

4. To assemble the taco muffins, put 1 tablespoon of the cornbread batter in the bottom of each prepared muffin cup (a cookie scoop works well) and spread with a wet finger to cover the bottom. Divide the filling among the cups (about 2 tablespoons in each) and top with an additional tablespoon of cornbread batter. Use a wet finger to spread and smooth out the surface of the muffin.

5. Bake for 20 minutes, until the cornbread is golden brown on top. Let cool for 10 minutes, then remove and serve.

KIDS CAN . . .

✳ Collect ingredients from the pantry and refrigerator

✳ Use a can opener to open the canned items (with supervision)

✳ Measure seasonings and put in a small bowl

✳ Measure wet and dry ingredients for the cornbread

✳ Put ingredients in the mixing bowls

✳ Mix ingredients with a whisk

✳ Help assemble the muffins

VARIATION

TRADITIONAL CORNBREAD: To make a loaf of regular cornbread, prepare the cornbread batter but omit the cheese. Bake in a greased 9 x 9-inch (23 x 23 cm) baking pan at 425°F (220°C) for 20 minutes.

 To make this recipe . . . .

DAIRY/LACTOSE/CASEIN-FREE

● Substitute canned unsweetened coconut milk for the cow's milk.

● Substitute melted coconut oil for the butter.

● Omit the cheese.

● If the batter is too thick, add up to an additional ½ cup coconut milk.

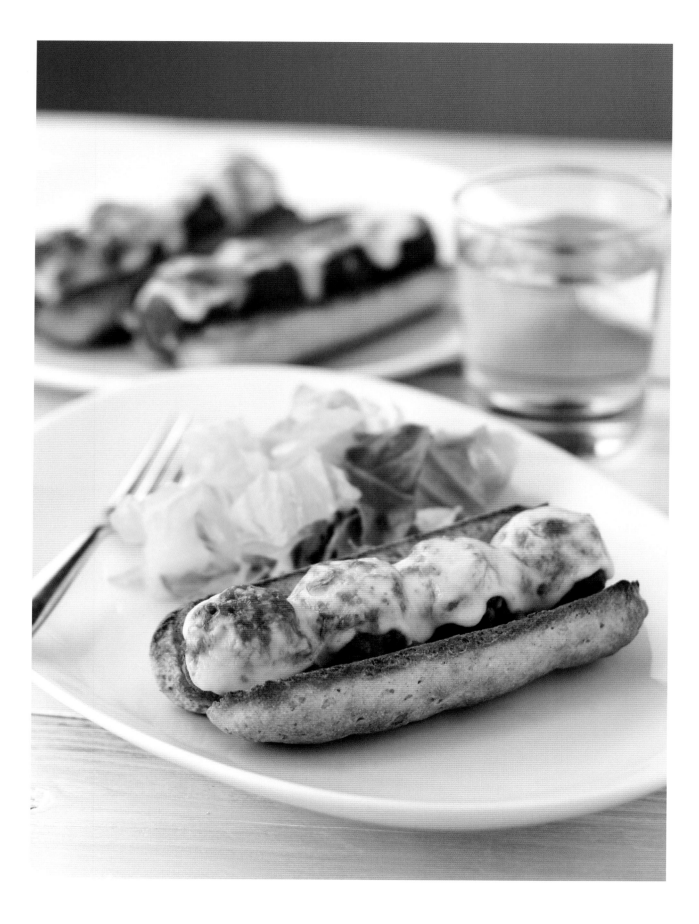

ITALIAN MEATBALL SUBS

• MAKES 4 SUB SANDWICHES •

Whether you call them subs, hoagies, grinders, or heroes, everyone should have a chance to enjoy this American staple. For our money, an Italian meatball sub is the way to go—topped with warm marinara sauce and melted mozzarella cheese. Of course, you can always pair the meatballs with some gluten-free spaghetti or Spaghetti Squash "Pasta" (page 92), or serve them on skewers like lollipops.

ROLLS

1 cup (240 ml) warm water

1 tablespoon sugar

2¼ teaspoons (1 packet) yeast

1 tablespoon olive oil

1⅓ cups plus 1 heaping tablespoon (175 g) Artisan GF Flour Blend (page 27)

1 teaspoon xanthan gum

¾ teaspoon salt

MEATBALLS

½ pound (227 g) ground turkey (93% lean)

1 egg

⅔ cup (79 g) GF bread crumbs (see page 75 to make your own)

¼ medium onion, diced fine

1 teaspoon dried basil

¾ teaspoon dried oregano

½ teaspoon garlic powder

½ teaspoon salt

½ teaspoon pepper

Olive oil

½ to ¾ cup (120 to 180 ml) Marinara Sauce (page 92)

4 slices mozzarella cheese, each cut in half (8 strips total)

KIDS CAN . . .

* Collect ingredients from the pantry and refrigerator

* Measure the ingredients

* Crack the egg

* Place the ingredients in the mixing bowl

* Mix ingredients with hands

* Shape meatballs

* Spoon the marinara sauce over the subs

* Place the slices of cheese on the subs

1. To make the rolls, combine the water, sugar, and yeast in a bowl and allow the mixture to rest for 5 minutes, until the yeast is active and the mixture bubbly with a layer of foam on top. Then add the olive oil.

2. In a separate bowl, whisk together the flour, xanthan gum, and salt. Pour the yeast mixture into the whisked flour mixture and mix to form a soft, wet dough.

3. Transfer the dough to a large zip-top bag and cut a corner off the bottom to make a slit that is 1¼ inches (3 cm) long. Pipe the dough to evenly divide among 4 slots of a hot dog bun pan.* Let rise in a warm place for 45 minutes.

4. Preheat the oven to 375°F (190°C). Bake the buns for 25 minutes, until golden brown on top.**

5. To make the meatballs, preheat the oven to 350°F/175°C; or, if you just baked the rolls, reduce the temperature to 350°F (175°C).

(RECIPE CONTINUES)

6. Combine the turkey, egg, bread crumbs, onion, basil, oregano, garlic powder, salt, and pepper in a large bowl. Mix thoroughly with your hands. Coat your hands in olive oil and form into 16 meatballs slightly smaller than a golf ball. Place the meatballs on an ungreased rimmed baking sheet. Bake for 20 minutes, until cooked through.***

7. To assemble the subs: Preheat the broiler. Slice the rolls almost in half lengthwise and place 4 meatballs in each. Spoon 2 to 3 tablespoons marinara sauce over each sub and top with 2 strips of sliced mozzarella cheese. Place under the broiler and watch carefully, removing when the cheese is melted and starting to brown, 2 to 3 minutes.

*If you do not have a hot dog pan, use 2 bread loaf pans and parchment paper: cut 4 pieces of parchment each 7 inches (18 cm) by the length of the bottom of your loaf pans. Pipe the dough down the center of each piece of parchment, then lift by the edges and transfer 2 tubes of dough—in their parchment—to each loaf pan. Let rise and bake as per the recipe.

**The rolls can be made ahead and frozen for later use. To reheat, pop in a 350°F (175°C) oven until warm, or microwave (times vary based on microwave strength; watch carefully).

***To add a richer flavor to the meatballs, first brown in a skillet over medium-high heat with 1 to 2 tablespoons olive oil, then finish cooking them through in the preheated oven, reducing the bake time to 15 minutes.

NOTE: The **refined-sugar-free**, **corn-free**, and **dairy/lactose/casein-free** statuses of this recipe are partially dependent on the ingredients in your bread crumbs. Our Sandwich Bread (page 80) can be made any combination of the above.

To make this recipe ....

DAIRY/LACTOSE/CASEIN-FREE
- In addition to confirming the bread status, omit the mozzarella cheese or substitute nondairy cheese.

CORN-FREE
- Use arrowroot flour to make a corn-free version of the Artisan GF Flour blend (page 26).

TURKEY BURGERS ON POTATO ROLLS

• MAKES 8 BURGERS •

Whether you opt for lean ground turkey as we do here, ground beef patties, or any other type of patty–veggie or otherwise–eating a proper burger on a potato roll will be a treat. Too many store-bought gluten-free hamburger buns are dry, white, starchy things that disintegrate in your hands as you try to eat your burger. The potato rolls for these turkey burgers, on the other hand, are chewy, moist, and easily hold together right through your last bite. Extra buns can also serve as great sandwich rolls.

POTATO ROLLS

1½ cups (355 ml) warm water

2 tablespoons sugar

1 tablespoon yeast

¼ cup (½ stick, 56 g) butter, melted

3 egg yolks

4½ tablespoons (50 g) potato flour

2 cups (250 g) Artisan GF Flour Blend (page 27)

½ teaspoon xanthan gum

⅓ cup (25 g) milk powder

1 teaspoon salt

BURGERS

2 pounds (907 g) ground turkey

Salt and pepper

8 slices American cheese, optional

KIDS CAN . . .

✳ Collect ingredients from the pantry and refrigerator

✳ Measure ingredients

✳ Put ingredients in the mixing bowl

✳ Crack eggs and separate egg yolks from whites

✳ Turn mixer on/off

✳ Roll the dough into balls

1. To make the rolls, combine the water, sugar, and yeast in the bowl of a stand mixer* and allow the mixture to rest for 5 minutes, until the yeast is active and the mixture bubbly with a layer of foam on top. Add the melted butter and egg yolks and mix to incorporate.

2. In a separate bowl, whisk together the potato flour, flour blend, xanthan gum, milk powder, and salt. With the paddle attachment mixing on medium-low, add the dry ingredients a bit at a time to the yeast mixture until fully incorporated. Mix for about 1 minute on medium. Scrape down the sides of the bowl.

3. Grease the cups of a hamburger bun pan or place eight 3½- to 4-inch (9 to 10 cm) greased rings (English muffin rings or tuna fish cans with both ends cut off) on a greased baking sheet.

4. Coat the palms of your hands liberally with olive oil, then pinch off a piece of dough that is about halfway between the size of a golf ball and a tennis ball (about 3½ ounces/100 g). Roll between your palms to make a perfectly smooth ball of dough.

5. Place the ball into one of the hamburger pan slots or greased rings and pat down gently, until the dough is flat and fills the full area of the cup or ring.

6. Repeat with the remaining dough.

(RECIPE CONTINUES)

To make this recipe . . . .

EGG-FREE
- In a small bowl combine 1 tablespoon ground flaxseeds and 3 tablespoons water. Allow the mixture to set for at least 2 minutes and use in place of the egg yolks.

DAIRY/LACTOSE/CASEIN-FREE:
- Substitute melted vegan shortening for the butter.
- Substitute ¼ cup (25 g) soy milk powder for the milk powder.

CORN-FREE
- Use arrowroot flour to make a corn-free version of the Artisan GF Flour Blend (page 26).

REFINED-SUGAR-FREE
- Substitute honey for the sugar to activate the yeast.

7. Cover the pan and let the dough rise in a warm location for 30 minutes, until doubled in size.

8. Preheat the oven to 350°F (175°C).

9. Bake the rolls for 20 minutes, until golden brown on top. Let cool on a wire rack.

10. To make the burgers, preheat a grill. Season the ground turkey with salt and pepper and form into 8 patties. Grill over medium-high heat until cooked through. If making cheeseburgers, place 1 piece of cheese on each cooked burger near the end of grilling time.

11. Slice the rolls in half, and serve each burger on a roll.

*To make the dough by hand (instead of using a stand mixer), start by adding only 1½ cups (188 g) of the flour, making sure to stir the dough until it is very smooth and sticky. Add up to ½ cup (63 g) additional flour if needed to work with the dough. The olive oil on your hands will enable you to shape and handle the dough even if it seems wet.

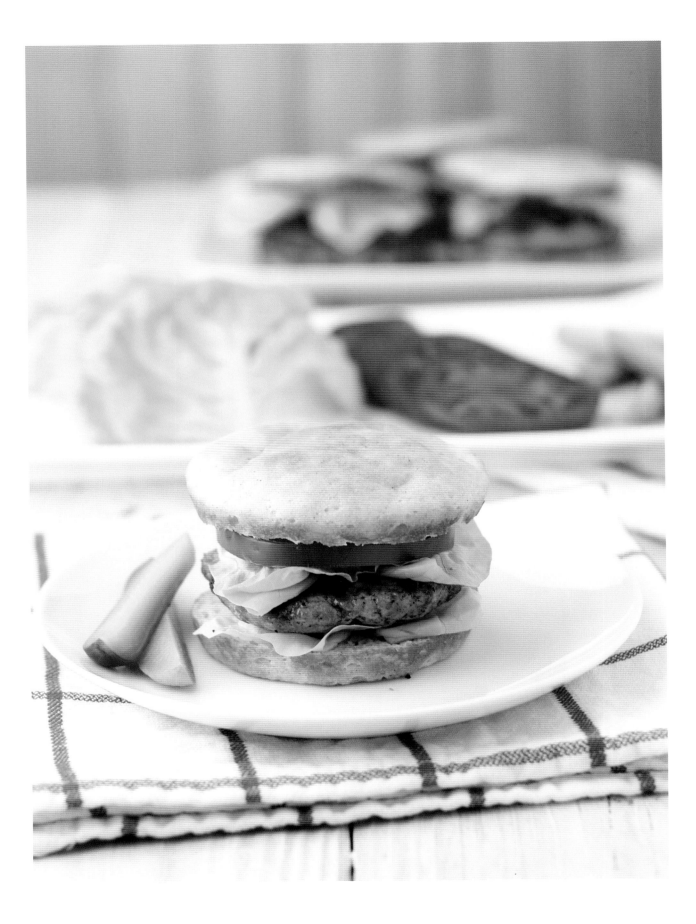

QUINOA MEATLOAF

• MAKES ONE 8 X 4-INCH (20 X 40 CM) LOAF •

This is turkey meatloaf transformed from ordinary to extraordinary with the use of quinoa as the binding agent (instead of bread crumbs), and the addition of bacon and raisins for moisture and richness. Using a food processor makes the prep quick and easy.

¼ cup (44 g) quinoa, rinsed in a fine-mesh strainer

½ cup (120 ml) GF low-sodium chicken broth or stock

½ medium onion, chopped

1 celery stalk, chopped

1 carrot, chopped

2 garlic cloves, peeled

1 tablespoon butter

1 tablespoon olive oil

1 tablespoon GF Worcestershire sauce

1½ teaspoons apple cider vinegar

½ teaspoon dried thyme

¼ teaspoon dried rubbed sage

¼ teaspoon chili powder

½ teaspoon salt

½ teaspoon pepper

5 shakes GF hot sauce

3 slices bacon, cut into pieces

¼ cup (38 g) raisins, loosely packed

1¼ pounds (567 g) ground turkey (93% lean)

1 egg

1. Combine the rinsed quinoa and chicken broth in a small saucepan over high heat and bring to a boil. Turn the heat down to low and simmer for 12 to 15 minutes, until the quinoa is translucent and tender and the liquid is absorbed. Set aside and let cool.

2. Preheat the oven to 350°F (175°C).

3. In a food processor, combine the onion, celery, carrot, and garlic and pulse until the vegetables are diced, but not a paste. Heat the butter and olive oil in a large skillet over medium-high heat. Add the finely diced vegetables and cook until the onion is translucent and soft, about 6 minutes.* Remove the vegetables from the heat and add the Worcestershire sauce, vinegar, thyme, sage, chili powder, salt, pepper, and hot sauce. Stir to combine.

4. In the food processor that chopped the vegetables, combine the bacon and raisins. Pulse until a paste is formed.

5. In a large bowl, combine the quinoa, vegetable mixture, bacon mixture, ground turkey, and egg and mix thoroughly with your hands. Place the mixture in a 9 x 9-inch (23 x 23 cm) pan and shape into an 8 x 4-inch (20 x 40 cm) loaf diagonally in the pan. Bake for 40 to 45 minutes, until the internal temperature is 160°F (70°C).

*To save time, omit the olive oil and butter and skip sautéing the vegetables.

KIDS CAN . . .

✳ Collect ingredients from the pantry and refrigerator

✳ Measure ingredients

✳ Add the vegetables to the food processor

✳ Press the food processor buttons

✳ Crack the egg

✳ Mix all of the ingredients with hands

To make this recipe. . . . .

EGG-FREE
● Omit the egg.

FISH-FREE
● Omit the Worcestershire sauce, which often contains anchovies.

DAIRY/LACTOSE/CASEIN-FREE
● Omit the butter and increase the olive oil to 2 tablespoons.

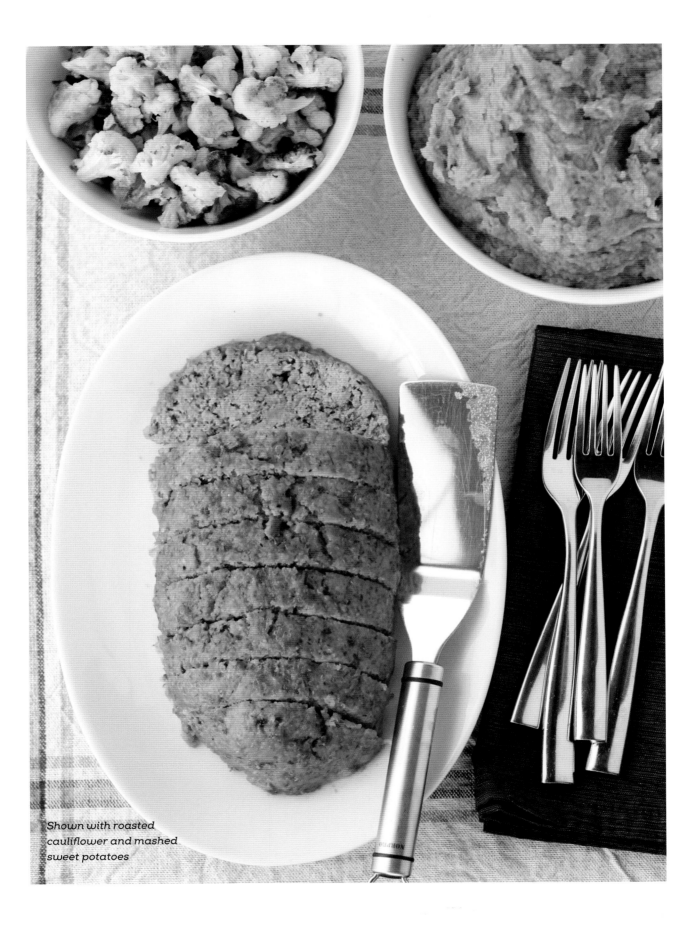

Shown with roasted cauliflower and mashed sweet potatoes

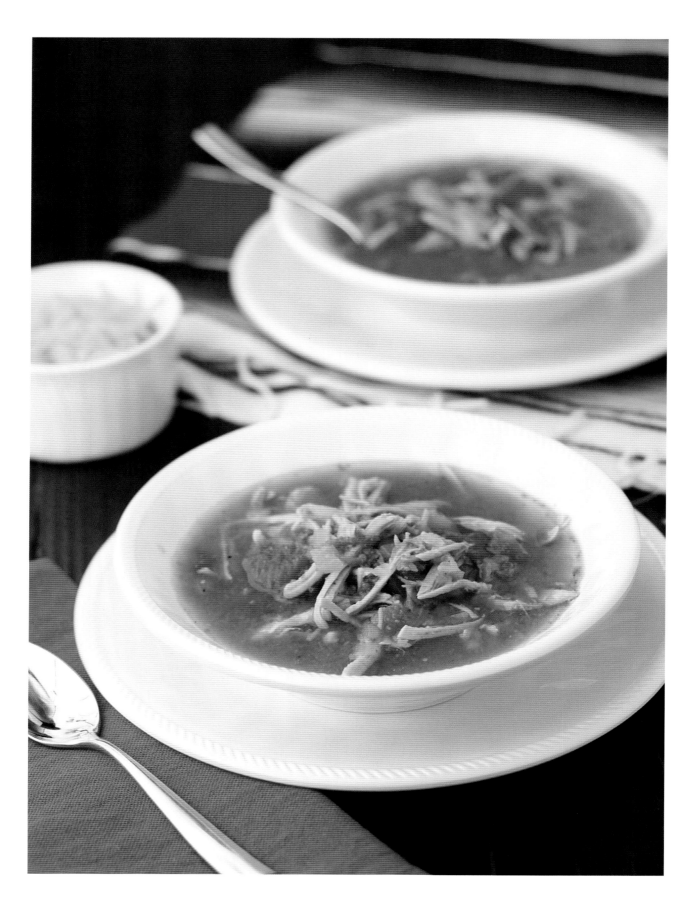

SLOW COOKER GREEN CHILI WITH PORK

• MAKES 6 TO 8 SERVINGS •

This slow-cooker chili—a great weeknight meal—is not too spicy, making it friendly for young mouths. We love to pair it with gluten-free cornbread, like the cornbread recipe that accompanies Cornbread Taco Muffins (page 135).

4 cups (945 ml) GF low-sodium chicken broth or stock

1½ cups (411 g) diced tomatoes or one 14.5-ounce (411 g) can no-salt-added diced tomatoes

One 7-ounce (200 g) can mild, fire-roasted, diced green chiles

1 medium yellow onion, diced

3 tomatillos, husked and diced

1 tablespoon ground cumin

1 tablespoon dried oregano

2 teaspoons garlic powder

1½ to 2 pounds (680 to 907 g) pork roast

Shredded cheddar cheese for serving, optional

Sour cream for serving, optional

1. In a slow cooker, combine the broth, tomatoes, chiles, onion, tomatillos, cumin, oregano, and garlic powder. Add the pork, cover, and cook on low for 8 to 10 hours.

2. Remove the roast and allow to cool. When it is cool enough to handle, shred the meat, discarding any fat pieces. Return the meat to the chili in the slow cooker. Serve, topping with cheese and sour cream if desired.

KIDS CAN . . .

* Collect ingredients from the pantry and refrigerator

* Dice tomatillos with age-appropriate knife

* Open chiles with the can opener (with supervision)

* Measure ingredients

* Put ingredients in the slow cooker

To make this recipe . . . .

DAIRY/LACTOSE/CASEIN-FREE

● Omit the cheese and sour cream, or use nondairy versions.

SPAGHETTI BOLOGNESE

• MAKES 6 TO 8 SERVINGS •

Families, gluten-free or not, often need quick weeknight meals. But every family also needs a long-stewing weekend dinner that fills the house with rich aromas on a Sunday afternoon into early evening. For us, the hearty meat sauce of this spaghetti Bolognese fits the bill. It's rich in iron and, just as importantly, kids gobble it down like Lady and the Tramp in the Disney classic.

2 small onions, quartered

2 small carrots, quartered

2 celery stalks, cut into segments

2 garlic cloves, peeled

2 tablespoons olive oil

1 pound (454 g) ground beef

½ teaspoon salt

One 6-ounce (170 g) can tomato paste

1 cup (240 ml) red wine*

1 cup (240 ml) water

1½ cups (411 g) diced tomatoes, or one 14.5-ounce can no-salt-added diced tomatoes

1 tablespoon dried basil

1 tablespoon dried oregano

1 pound (454 g) GF spaghetti

Parmesan cheese, optional

KIDS CAN . . .

∗ Collect ingredients from the pantry and refrigerator

∗ Add the vegetables to the food processor

∗ Press the food processor buttons

∗ Measure the ingredients

∗ Place ingredients into saucepan

1. Place the onions, carrots, celery, and garlic in the food processor and pulse until finely chopped, almost a paste.

2. Heat the olive oil in a large saucepan over medium-high heat. Add the vegetables from the food processor and sauté, stirring regularly, for 20 minutes, until very soft and slightly brown. Add the beef and salt. Continue to cook over medium-high heat, stirring frequently, for about 15 minutes, until the meat is very brown. When stirring, make sure to scrape up all the little brown bits stuck to the bottom of the pan. Add the tomato paste, turn the heat down to medium, and cook for 5 minutes, stirring frequently. Add the red wine and water and cook for 5 more minutes.

3. Puree the diced tomatoes in the food processor. Add to the beef mixture along with the basil and oregano. Reduce the heat to just a simmer and cook for 30 minutes, stirring occasionally, until the sauce is very thick and dark.

4. While the sauce is simmering, cook the spaghetti in a large pot of salted boiling water until al dente,

5. Drain the spaghetti and add to the sauce, along with a little pasta water if the sauce is too thick. Serve with freshly grated Parmesan if desired.

*If you're concerned about the red wine in this kid's dish, don't be. The alcohol burns off long before it ever makes it to their plates. Alternatively, replace the 1 cup wine with 1 cup GF low-sodium beef broth or stock or an additional 1 cup water.

To make this recipe . . . .

CORN-FREE

• Check to make sure you're using corn-free gluten-free spaghetti, such as that made from brown rice or quinoa.

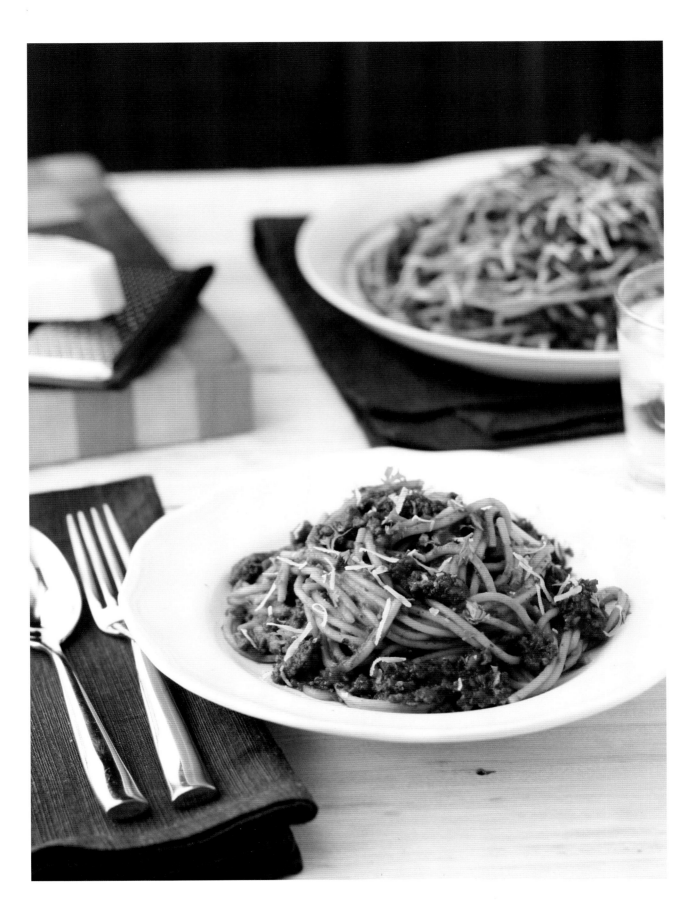

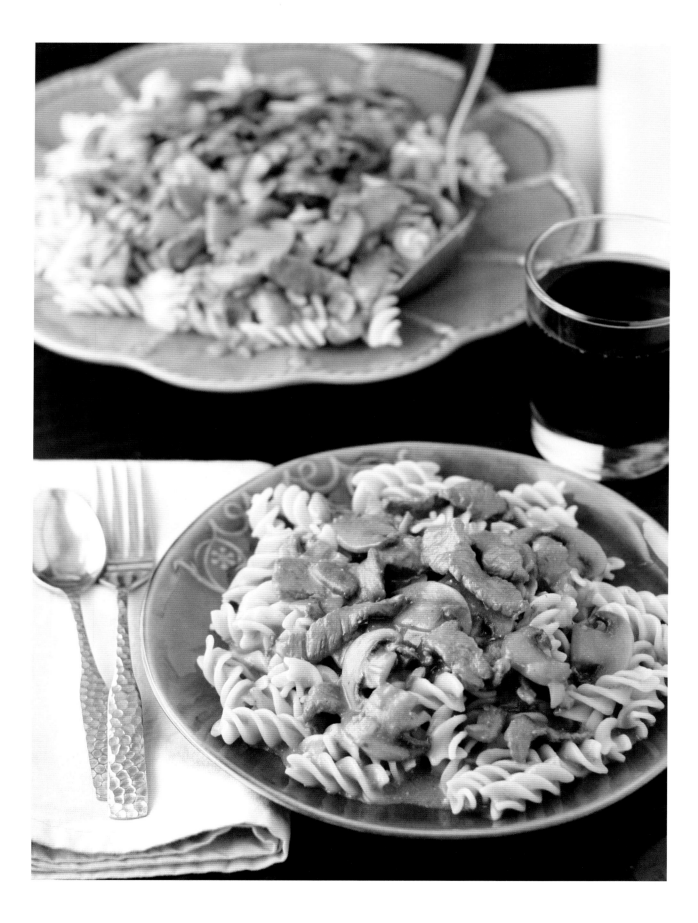

BEEF STROGANOFF

• MAKES 4 SERVINGS •

This version of beef stroganoff starts with making a delicious sauce filled with tender pieces of beef and mushrooms and finished, if you like, with a dollop of sour cream. We enjoy the stroganoff best over noodles.

3 tablespoons butter

1 pound (454 g) beef (e.g., top sirloin steak), cut into thin slices

1½ teaspoons olive oil

1 medium onion, diced small

1 pound (454 g) mushrooms, sliced

1½ cups (355 ml) GF low-sodium beef broth or stock

½ cup (120 ml) white wine*

2 tablespoons Artisan GF Flour Blend (page 27)

2 to 4 tablespoons sour cream, optional

KIDS CAN...

* Collect ingredients from the pantry and refrigerator

* Cut the mushrooms with age-appropriate knife

* Measure the liquid ingredients

* Place ingredients into pan

1. Heat a large skillet or sauté pan over medium-high heat. Add 1 tablespoon of the butter and the beef and sauté until the meat is browned and all of the liquid has evaporated. Remove the meat from the pan and set aside.

2. Heat the remaining 2 tablespoons butter and the olive oil in the pan. Add the diced onion and sauté for about 1 minute, until softened. Add the mushrooms and sauté for about 3 minutes, until softened.

3. In a small bowl, whisk together the broth, wine, and flour. Return the beef to the pan and add the broth mixture, stirring to combine. When the mixture comes to a simmer, turn the heat down to low and continue to simmer for about 30 minutes, stirring occasionally, until the sauce is thick and the meat is tender.

4. Remove from the heat and stir in the sour cream, if desired. Serve over gluten-free pasta or rice, if desired.

*If you're concerned about the white wine in this kid's dish, don't be. The alcohol burns off long before it ever makes it to their plates. Alternatively, replace the ½ cup wine with an additional ½ cup GF low-sodium beef broth or stock.

To make this recipe..

DAIRY/LACTOSE/CASEIN-FREE
* Substitute olive oil for the butter.
* Substitute nondairy sour cream for the dairy sour cream.

CORN-FREE
* Use arrowroot flour to make a corn-free version of the Artisan GF Flour Blend (page 26).

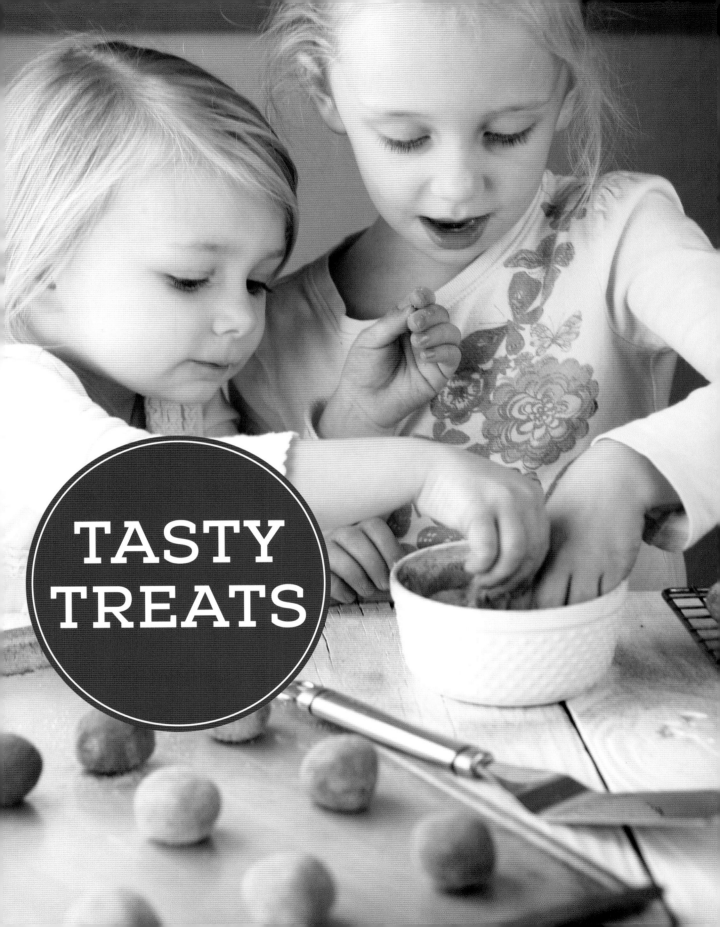

TASTY
TREATS

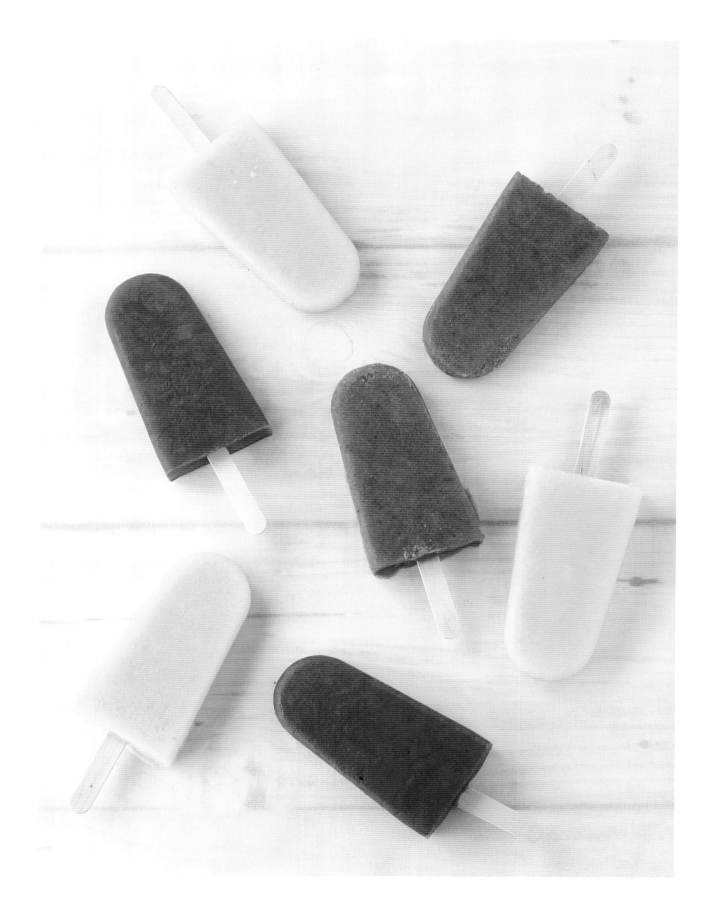

FROZEN FRUIT POPS

It doesn't get much simpler than fresh fruit, a little lemon juice to brighten the flavor, and maybe a wee bit of sweetener for tart fruit. These frozen fruit pops are nothing but pure, natural ingredients you can feel good about your kids eating.

2 cups chopped fruit (e.g., 360 g peaches, 340 g mangos, 280 g berries)

Juice of ½ lemon (about 2 tablespoons)

2 to 3 tablespoons agave nectar, if needed, depending on sweetness of the fruit

1. Place the fruit and lemon juice in the food processor and blend until smooth.* Add agave nectar to taste.

2. Pour the fruit puree into ice pop molds and freeze for at least 4 hours.

3. Remove the pops from the molds and serve or place in a heavy-duty zip-top bag and keep in the freezer.

*If your kids do not like "pieces" in their pops, strain the puree through a fine mesh strainer to catch bits of seeds and skins.

KIDS CAN . . .

✳ Collect ingredients from the pantry and refrigerator

✳ Help cut up fruit with age-appropriate knife

✳ Measure ingredients

✳ Juice the lemon using a citrus reamer over a strainer to catch the seeds

✳ Dump ingredients into food processor

✳ Press the food processor buttons

LEMON BARS

• MAKES 16 BARS •

Cashews help form the base for these lemon bars, while plenty of fresh-squeezed lemon juice makes them burst with bright flavor. Honey and brown sugar help balance the zing of the lemons, making the bars a little sweet and a little tart.

CRUST

½ cup (74 g) raw cashew pieces

1 cup (125 g) Artisan GF Flour Blend (page 27)

¼ cup (58 g) packed light brown sugar

¼ teaspoon salt

6 tablespoons (¾ stick, 84 g) butter

½ teaspoon GF pure vanilla extract

FILLING

4 eggs

½ cup (170 g) honey

6 tablespoons (46 g) Artisan GF Flour Blend

Zest of 2 lemons

½ cup (120 ml) fresh lemon juice (2 to 4 lemons)

½ cup (115 g) packed light brown sugar*

Confectioners' sugar (see below to make your own)

1. Preheat the oven to 350°F (175°C). Grease a 9 x 9-inch (23 x 23 cm) pan with butter or nonstick cooking spray.

2. To make the crust, pulse the cashew pieces in the food processor into fine crumbs. Add the flour, sugar, and salt and pulse to combine. Add the butter and vanilla and pulse until a dough forms. Press the dough into an even layer in the prepared pan, using a piece of plastic wrap or parchment paper on your hand if the dough is too sticky.

3. Bake for 20 minutes until the crust is golden brown. Set aside.

4. To make the filling, whisk together the eggs and honey in a bowl until smooth. Add the flour, lemon zest and juice, and brown sugar and whisk to combine.

5. Pour the lemon mixture over the baked crust. Return to the oven and bake for 20 to 25 minutes, until the filling is set. Let cool completely, then cut into bars. Sprinkle with confectioners' sugar right before serving. Refrigerate in an airtight container for up to 3 days.

*To knock back the tartness for a sweeter lemon bar, use an additional ¼ cup brown sugar in the filling.

Make your own . . .

CORN-FREE CONFECTIONERS' SUGAR: Combine 1 cup granulated sugar and 1 tablespoon tapioca starch in a blender and blend until uniformly powdery.

KIDS CAN . . .

* Collect ingredients from the pantry and refrigerator

* Measure ingredients

* Dump ingredients into the food processor and mixing bowl

* Press the food processor buttons

* Press the dough into the pan

* Crack the eggs

* Mix filling ingredients with a whisk

* Sprinkle confectioners' sugar on top

To make this recipe . . . .

DAIRY/LACTOSE/CASEIN-FREE

• Substitute melted coconut oil for the butter.

CORN-FREE

• Use arrowroot flour to make a corn-free version of the Artisan GF Flour Blend (page 26).

• Omit the confectioners' sugar, which typically contains cornstarch, or use a corn-free confectioners' sugar, such as those made with tapioca, or make your own (see below).

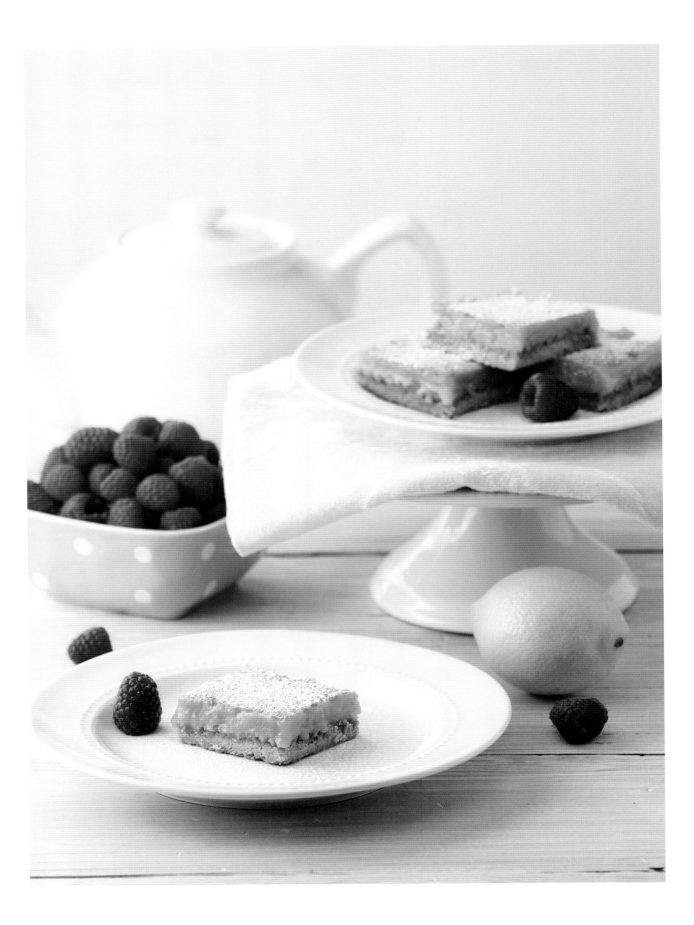

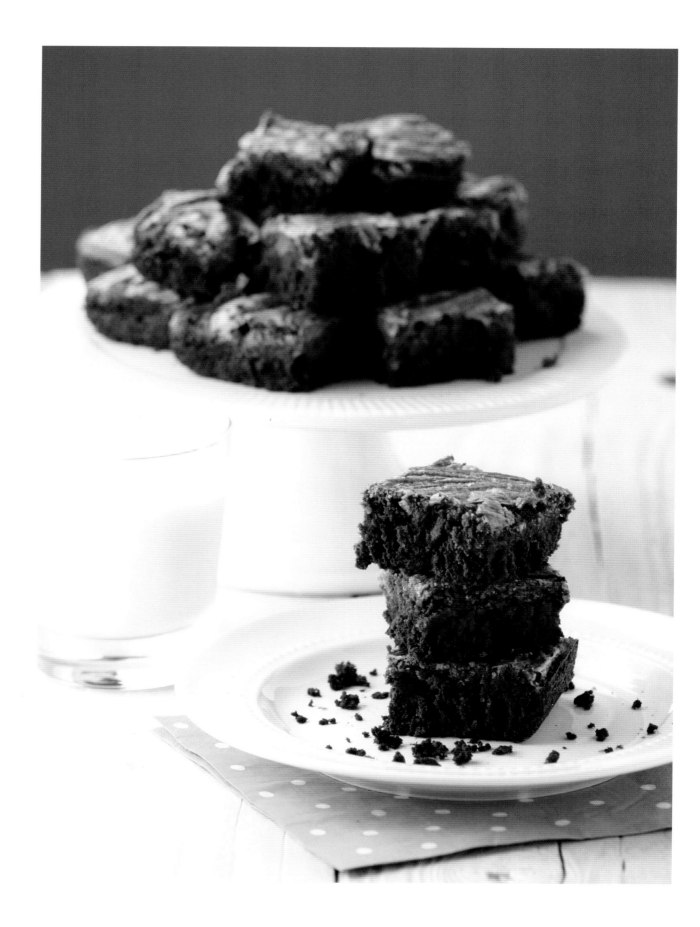

CHOCOLATE PEANUT BUTTER BROWNIES

• MAKES 16 BROWNIES •

Chocolate and peanut butter are a flavor marriage made in heaven. By swirling their respective brownie batters together, each retains its distinct qualities while playing off the other. The result is a moist, chewy brownie that's as fun for your kids to make as it is for them to eat.

CHOCOLATE BATTER

½ cup (1 stick, 113 g) butter

4 ounces (113 g) high-quality unsweetened chocolate, pieces or chopped

1 cup (230 g) packed brown sugar

2 eggs

1 teaspoon GF pure vanilla extract

½ cup (63 g) Artisan GF Flour Blend (page 27)

¼ teaspoon GF baking powder

PEANUT BUTTER BATTER

¼ cup (65 g) smooth/creamy peanut butter

3 tablespoons butter

½ cup (115 g) packed brown sugar

1 egg

½ teaspoon GF pure vanilla extract

6 tablespoons (46 g) Artisan GF Flour Blend

¼ teaspoon GF baking powder

KIDS CAN . . .

* Collect ingredients from the pantry and refrigerator

* Measure ingredients

* Crack the eggs

* Dump ingredients into the saucepans

* Mix filling ingredients with a spoon

* Swirl batters together

1. Preheat the oven to 350°F (175°C). Grease a 9 x 9-inch (23 x 23 cm) baking pan with butter or nonstick cooking spray.

2. To make the chocolate batter, melt the butter and chocolate in a saucepan over medium-low heat, stirring occasionally. Remove from the heat and stir in the brown sugar, eggs, and vanilla, mixing until smooth. Stir in the flour and baking powder until combined. Spread the batter in the prepared pan.

3. To make the peanut butter batter, melt the peanut butter and butter in a saucepan over medium-low heat, stirring occasionally. Remove from the heat and stir in the brown sugar, egg, and vanilla, mixing until smooth. Stir in the flour and baking powder until combined.

4. Drizzle the peanut butter batter on top of the chocolate batter. Using a butter knife, swirl the two batters together, resulting in a marbled look. Bake for 30 minutes, until the edges are set and a toothpick inserted in the middle comes out mostly clean. Cool, cut, and serve.

HIGH-ALTITUDE ADJUSTMENTS: Increase the flour in the chocolate batter to ½ cup plus 3 tablespoons (86 g). Increase the flour in the peanut butter batter to ½ cup (63 g).

To make this recipe . . . .

PEANUT-FREE
● Substitute sunflower seed butter for the peanut butter.

SOY-FREE
● Confirm that your chocolate does not contain soy lecithin.

EGG-FREE
● In a small bowl, combine 2 tablespoons ground flaxseeds and 6 tablespoons water. Allow the mixture to set for at least 2 minutes and use in place of the eggs in the chocolate brownies.
● Use 1 tablespoon ground flaxseeds and 3 tablespoons water in place of the egg in the peanut butter brownies.

DAIRY/LACTOSE/CASEIN-FREE
● Substitute melted coconut oil for the butter.

CORN-FREE
● Use arrowroot flour to make a corn-free version of the Artisan GF Flour Blend (page 26).
● Check the ingredients of your baking powder, which often contains cornstarch.

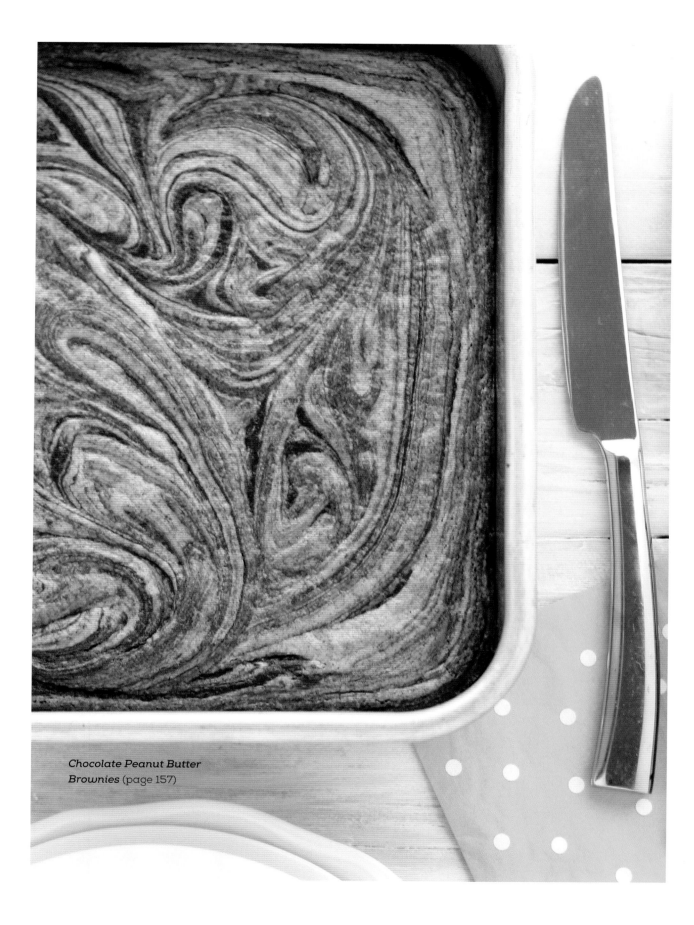

Chocolate Peanut Butter Brownies (page 157)

FIG EINSTEINS

• MAKES 36 COOKIES •

You've heard of the Fig Newton, Nabisco's classic treat—a flattened roll, with a fig paste filling contained inside a pastry that's somewhere between a cake and a cookie. Now meet our Fig Einstein, the Newton's gluten-free, made-from-scratch-at-home twin. Same great flavors and textures, minus the gluten.

FIG FILLING

1 cup (160 g) chopped, stemmed dried figs

1 cup (240 ml) orange juice

2 tablespoons honey

Zest of 1 lemon

DOUGH

1½ cups plus 2 tablespoons (204 g) Artisan GF Flour Blend (page 27)

1 teaspoon xanthan gum

¼ cup (54 g) sugar

½ teaspoon GF baking powder

¼ teaspoon baking soda

¼ teaspoon cinnamon

¼ teaspoon salt

6 tablespoons (¾ stick, 84 g) butter

2 eggs

1 teaspoon GF pure vanilla extract

KIDS CAN . . .

* Collect ingredients from the pantry and refrigerator

* Measure ingredients

* Crack the eggs

* Dump ingredients into the saucepan and bowls

* Mix ingredients with a spoon

* Spread the filling on each dough rectangle

1. To make the filling, combine all ingredients in a saucepan and bring to a simmer over medium heat. Simmer, stirring occasionally, until the liquid is absorbed and the mixture is thick, about 30 minutes. With either an immersion blender or conventional blender, puree the filling until fairly smooth. Refrigerate until cool.

2. To make the dough, combine the flour, xanthan gum, sugar, baking powder, baking soda, cinnamon, and salt in a large bowl and whisk to combine. Cut the butter into chunks and work it into the flour mixture with a pastry cutter or your hands until the mixture resembles sand. In a separate bowl, whisk together the eggs and vanilla. Add to the flour mixture and mix until dough forms.

3. Preheat the oven to 350°F (175°C). Line a baking sheet with parchment paper or a silicone mat.

4. Roll the dough out between two pieces of plastic wrap to form a rectangle about 18 x 10 inches (45 x 25 cm). Remove the top piece of plastic wrap and set aside. Use a pizza cutter or knife to cut the dough into 9 equal rectangles. (Make two evenly spaced vertical cuts and two evenly spaced horizontal cuts. You'll end up with rectangles about 6 x 3 inches/15 x 8 cm.)

5. Keeping the dough on the bottom piece of plastic wrap, slide onto another baking sheet and place in the refrigerator until the filling has finished cooling, about 10 minutes.

6. Remove the dough and fig filling from the refrigerator. Move one rectangle of dough to the reserved piece of plastic wrap and spread 1½ tablespoons of filling in a roughly 1-inch (2.5 cm) strip lengthwise down the center. Use the edge of the plastic wrap to lift one long side of the dough and fold over so the edge runs down

(RECIPE CONTINUES)

the middle. Repeat with the other long side to create a tube. Press to slightly flatten. Place the tube seam-side down on the prepared baking sheet. Repeat with the remaining dough and filling.

7. Bake for 10 to 12 minutes, until slightly golden Cut each roll crosswise into 4 pieces while still hot, and immediately place in a container with a lid, ideally in a single layer (or in multiple layers separated by sheets of parchment paper). This allows the Fig Einsteins to steam while cooling, resulting in the soft, cake-like texture of the rolls.

HIGH-ALTITUDE ADJUSTMENT: Increase the flour to 1¾ cups.

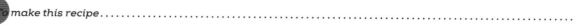

To make this recipe...

EGG-FREE

- In a small bowl, combine 2 tablespoons ground flaxseeds and 6 tablespoons water. Allow the mixture to set for at least 2 minutes and use in place of the eggs.

DAIRY/LACTOSE/CASEIN-FREE

- Substitute vegan shortening for the butter.

CORN-FREE

- Use arrowroot flour to make a corn-free version of the Artisan GF Flour Blend (page 26).
- Check the ingredients of your baking powder, which often contains cornstarch.

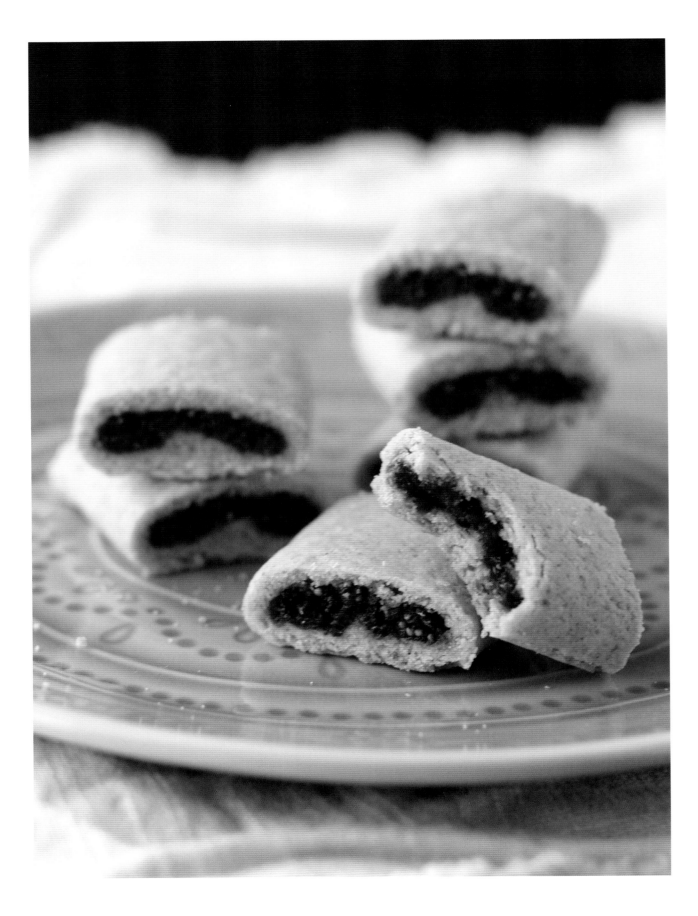

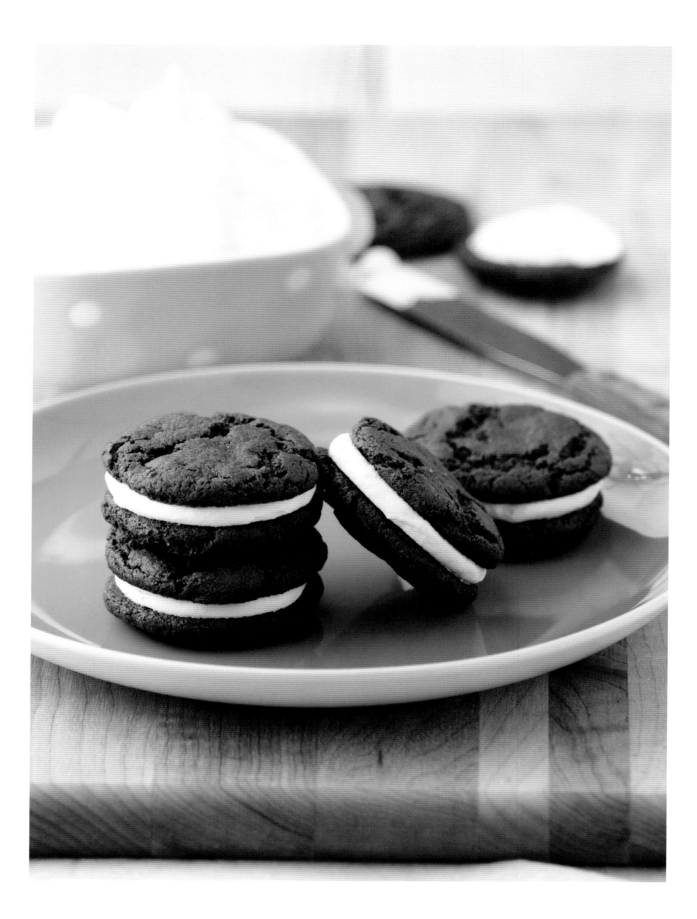

CHOCOLATE COOKIES WITH FLUFFY FROSTING

• MAKES 20 COOKIE SANDWICHES •

A marshmallow-like filling sandwiched between two small chocolate cookies offers up a play of textures and sweetness. Whether your children prefer the fluff, the cookie, or both, these are sure to please.

COOKIES

½ cup (1 stick, 113 g) butter, softened

½ cup (115 g) packed light brown sugar

¼ cup (54 g) granulated sugar

½ teaspoon GF pure vanilla extract

1 egg

¾ cup (94 g) Artisan GF Flour Blend (page 27)

1 teaspoon xanthan gum

½ teaspoon baking soda

½ cup (40 g) cocoa powder

¼ teaspoon salt

FROSTING

¾ cup (162 g) granulated sugar

3 tablespoons water

1 egg white

⅛ teaspoon cream of tartar

½ teaspoon GF pure vanilla extract

KIDS CAN . . .

＊ Collect ingredients from the pantry and refrigerator

＊ Measure ingredients

＊ Crack the egg

＊ Dump ingredients into the mixing bowl

＊ Turn the mixer on/off

＊ Whisk the dry ingredients

＊ Scoop the cookies onto the baking sheet

＊ Spread the frosting on the cookies and make the sandwiches

1. Preheat the oven to 375°F (190°C).

2. To make the cookies, cream together the butter, brown sugar, granulated sugar, and vanilla with a mixer on medium speed. Add the egg, mixing until incorporated. In a separate bowl, whisk together the flour, xanthan gum, baking soda, cocoa powder, and salt; add to the butter mixture and mix until well blended.

3. Shape the cookie dough into 1-teaspoon-size balls and place on ungreased baking sheets—or one sheet, baking in batches—1 inch (2.5 cm) apart. There should be 40 cookies. Bake for 7 minutes, until the cookies puff and are cracked on top. Let the cookies rest for 2 minutes, then transfer to a wire rack to cool completely.

4. While the cookies are cooling, make the frosting. Combine the granulated sugar, water, egg white, and cream of tartar in a metal or glass bowl. Use a handheld mixer to combine the ingredients. Place the bowl over a pot of simmering water to create a double boiler; the bottom of the bowl should not touch the water. Mix in the double boiler on high for 7 minutes, until the frosting is fluffy like marshmallow. Remove from the heat and mix in the vanilla. Beat on high for another 2 minutes

5. To assemble the cookies, spread frosting on the bottom side of one cookie and top with another cookie to create a sandwich. Repeat to make 20 cookie sandwiches.*

*The assembled cookies are best the first day. If you will not be eating them immediately, frost the cookies just before serving.

HIGH-ALTITUDE ADJUSTMENT: Increase the flour to 1 cup (125 g).

To make this recipe . . . .

DAIRY/LACTOSE/CASEIN-FREE
● Substitute vegan shortening for the butter.

CORN-FREE
● Use arrowroot flour to make a corn-free version of the Artisan GF Flour Blend (page 26).

PEANUT BUTTER COOKIES WITH CHOCOLATE CLOVERS

• MAKES 36 COOKIES •

These moist, chewy cookies pack a serious punch of peanut butter flavor, while the chocolate "prize" on top elevates them from plain old cookies to fun treat.

½ cup (1 stick, 113 g) butter

½ cup (130 g) smooth/creamy peanut butter

½ cup (108 g) granulated sugar, plus more for rolling the dough balls

½ cup (115 g) packed brown sugar

1 teaspoon GF pure vanilla extract

1 egg

1¼ cups (156 g) Artisan GF Flour Blend (page 27)

1 teaspoon xanthan gum

½ teaspoon baking soda

½ teaspoon GF baking powder

144 chocolate baking chips or chocolate chips (134 g)

1. Preheat the oven to 375°F (190°C).

2. Cream together the butter, peanut butter, granulated sugar, brown sugar, and vanilla with a mixer on medium speed. Add the egg and mix until combined. In a separate bowl, whisk together the flour, xanthan gum, baking soda, and baking powder; add to the butter mixture and mix to incorporate.

3. Shape the dough into 1-inch (2.5 cm) balls and roll in granulated sugar. Place the cookies 2 inches (5 cm) apart on ungreased baking sheets—or one sheet, baking in batches. Bake for 7 to 9 minutes, until lightly browned. Immediately press 4 chocolate chips into each cookie. Let rest on the baking sheet for 5 minutes. Transfer to a wire rack to cool completely.

HIGH-ALTITUDE ADJUSTMENT: Increase the flour to 1½ cups (188 g).

KIDS CAN...

* Collect ingredients from the pantry and refrigerator

* Measure ingredients

* Crack the egg

* Dump ingredients into the mixing bowl

* Turn the mixer on/off

* Whisk the dry ingredients

* Shape the dough balls, roll in sugar, and place on baking sheet

* Press the chocolate chips into the cookies

To make this recipe . . . .

PEANUT-FREE
- Substitute sunflower seed butter for the peanut butter.

SOY-FREE
- Confirm that your chocolate chips do not contain soy lecithin.

EGG-FREE
- In a small bowl, combine 1 tablespoon ground flaxseeds and 3 tablespoons water. Allow the mixture to set for at least 2 minutes and use in place of the egg.

DAIRY/LACTOSE/CASEIN-FREE
- Substitute vegan shortening for the butter.
- Confirm that your chocolate chips do not contain dairy.

CORN-FREE
- Use arrowroot flour to make a corn-free version of the Artisan GF Flour Blend (page 26).
- Check the ingredients of your baking powder, which often contains cornstarch.

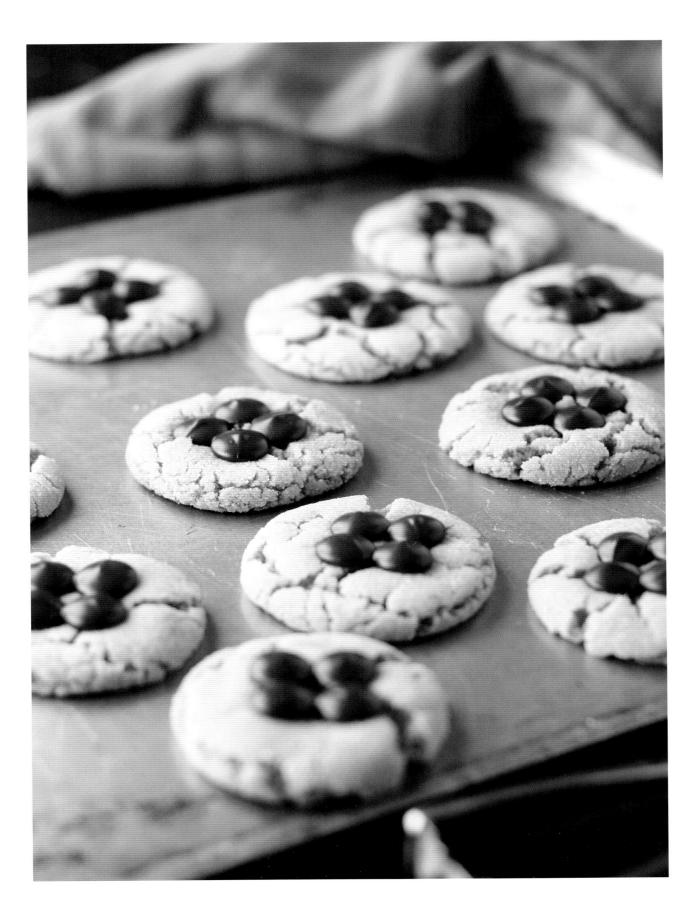

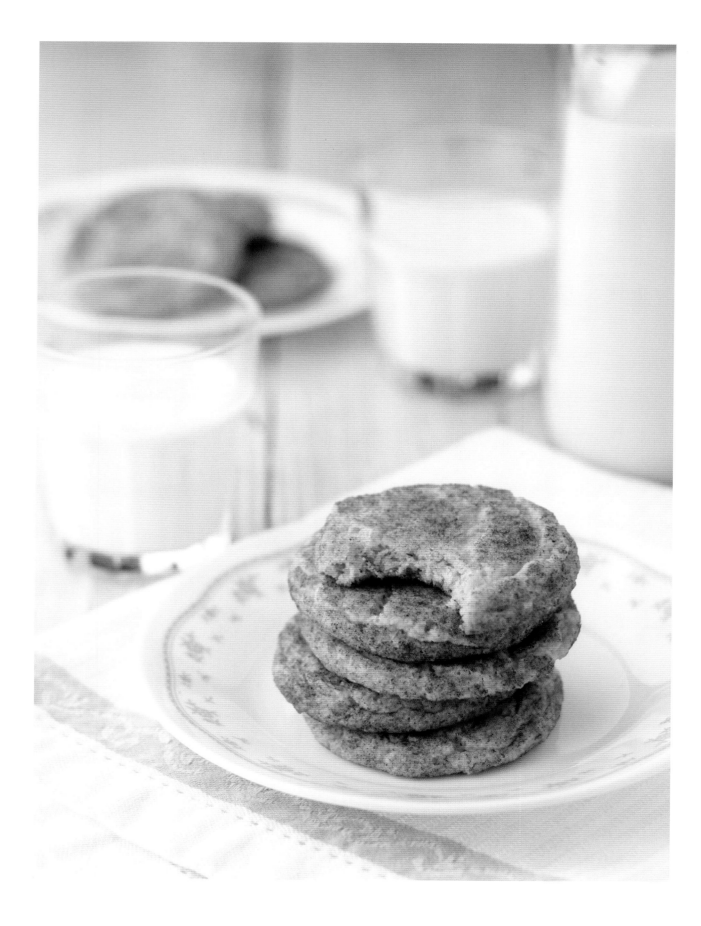

SNICKERDOODLES

• MAKES 45 COOKIES •

The cinnamon-sugar combo of snickerdoodle cookies is beloved by kids everywhere. And the process of rolling cookie dough balls in the cinnamon-sugar mix is just made for kids to help!

1½ cups (324 g) plus 2 tablespoons sugar

1 cup (2 sticks, 226 g) butter, softened

2 eggs

2½ cups (313 g) Artisan GF Flour Blend (page 27)

2 teaspoons xanthan gum

2 teaspoons cream of tartar

1 teaspoon baking soda

¼ teaspoon salt

2 teaspoons ground cinnamon

1. Preheat the oven to 400°F (205°C).

2. Cream together 1½ cups of the sugar and the butter with a mixer on medium speed until light and fluffy. Add the eggs and mix until incorporated. In a separate bowl, whisk together the flour, xanthan gum, cream of tartar, baking soda, and salt. Add to the butter-sugar mixture and mix to incorporate.

3. Mix together the remaining 2 tablespoons sugar and the cinnamon in a small bowl.

4. Shape the dough into 1-tablespoon-size balls and roll in the cinnamon sugar. Place the balls 2 inches (5 cm) apart on ungreased baking sheets—or one sheet, baking in batches—and gently flatten with the palm of your hand. Bake for 8 to 10 minutes, until slightly brown at the edges. Let rest on the baking sheet for 5 minutes. Transfer to a wire rack to cool completely.

HIGH-ALTITUDE ADJUSTMENTS: Increase the flour to 3 cups (375 g) and do not flatten the cookies before baking.

KIDS CAN . . .

* Collect ingredients from the pantry and refrigerator

* Measure ingredients

* Crack the eggs

* Dump ingredients into the mixing bowl

* Turn the mixer on/off

* Whisk the dry ingredients

* Shape the dough balls, roll in the cinnamon sugar, and place on baking sheet

To make this recipe . . . .

EGG-FREE
- In a small bowl, combine 2 tablespoons ground flaxseeds and 6 tablespoons water. Allow the mixture to set for at least 2 minutes and use in place of the eggs.

DAIRY/LACTOSE/CASEIN-FREE
- Substitute vegan shortening for the butter.
- Add 1 teaspoon GF pure vanilla extract with the eggs.

CORN-FREE
- Use arrowroot flour to make a corn-free version of the Artisan GF Flour Blend (page 26).

CHOCOLATE CHIP COOKIES

• MAKES 40 COOKIES •

This cookie staple is chewy in all the right ways, and we'd bet your kids and their friends won't be able to tell they're gluten-free. That's no small claim, especially since a classic cookie such as this has the burden of needing to "compete" with familiar and beloved glutenous versions. But go right ahead: Leave these out on a plate for Santa on Christmas Eve. He'll approve.

1 cup (2 sticks, 226 g) butter, softened

¾ cup (173 g) packed light brown sugar

¾ cup (162 g) granulated sugar

1 teaspoon GF pure vanilla extract

2 eggs

2¼ cups (281 g) Artisan GF Flour Blend (page 27)

2 teaspoons xanthan gum

1 teaspoon baking soda

½ teaspoon salt

10 ounces (1⅔ cups, 283 g) chocolate chips

1. Preheat the oven to 375°F (190°C).

2. Cream together the butter, brown sugar, granulated sugar, and vanilla with a mixer on medium speed, about 2 minutes. Add the eggs one at a time, mixing until incorporated. In a separate bowl, whisk together the flour, xanthan gum, baking soda, and salt. Add to the butter mixture and mix until blended. Mix in the chocolate chips.

3. Shape the cookie dough into 1-tablespoon-size balls and place on ungreased baking sheets—or one sheet, baking in batches—2 inches (5 cm) apart. Bake for 8 to 10 minutes, until lightly golden on top. Let the cookies rest for 5 minutes on the baking sheet. Transfer to a wire rack to cool.

HIGH-ALTITUDE ADJUSTMENT: Increase the flour to 2¾ cups (344 g).

KIDS CAN . . .

* Collect ingredients from the pantry and refrigerator

* Measure ingredients

* Crack the eggs

* Dump ingredients into the mixing bowl

* Turn the mixer on/off

* Whisk the dry ingredients

* Shape the cookies and place on the baking sheet

To make this recipe. . . . .

SOY-FREE

● Confirm that your chocolate chips do not contain soy lecithin.

EGG-FREE

● In a small bowl, combine 2 tablespoons ground flaxseeds and 6 tablespoons water. Allow the mixture to set for at least 2 minutes and use in place of the eggs.

DAIRY/LACTOSE/CASEIN-FREE

● Substitute vegan shortening for the butter.

● Confirm that your chocolate chips do not contain dairy.

CORN-FREE

● Use arrowroot flour to make a corn-free version of the Artisan GF Flour Blend (page 26).

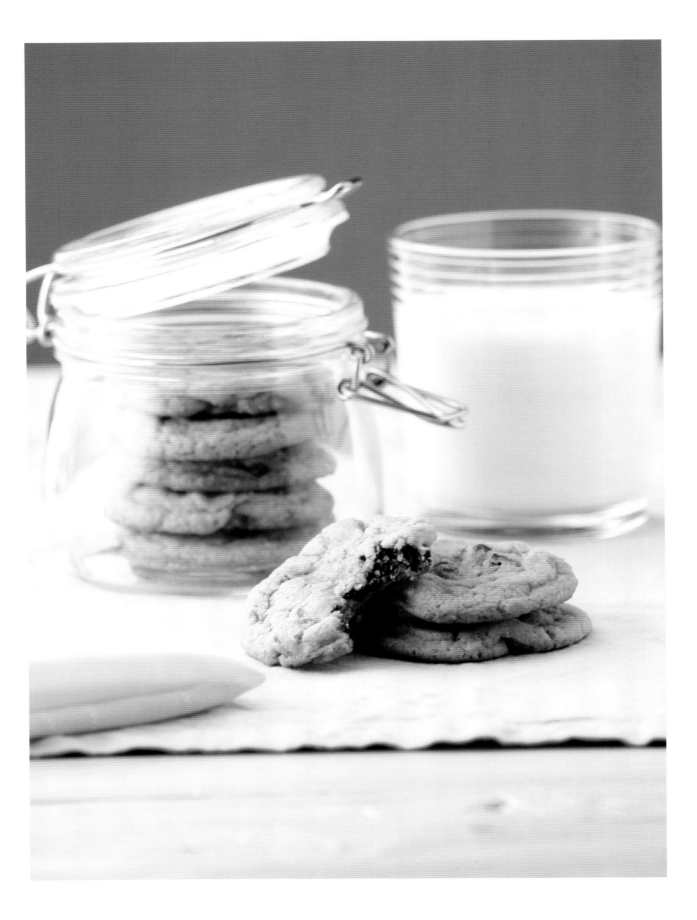

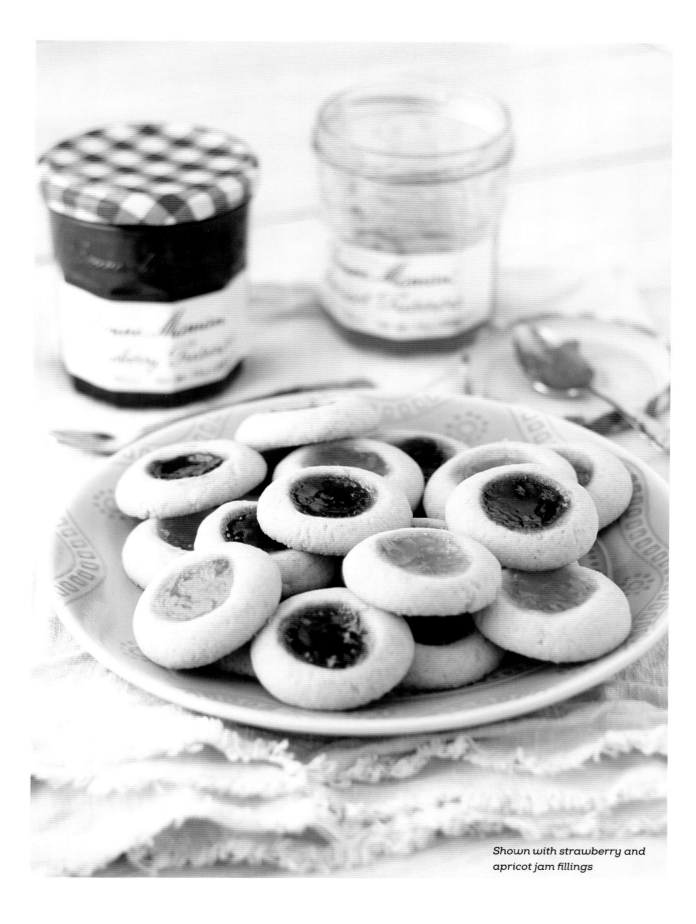

Shown with strawberry and apricot jam fillings

THUMBPRINT JAM COOKIES

It's often tempting for little hands and fingers to find their way into your kitchen work and create all sorts of dents and divots in doughs and cakes and such. With these thumbprint cookies, you can give your kids license to press that dough and make some craters. Then fill the craters with dollops of your favorite jam!

½ cup (1 stick, 113 g) butter

¼ cup (54 g) sugar

1 egg yolk

1 teaspoon GF pure vanilla extract

1 cup (125 g) Artisan GF Flour Blend (page 27)

¼ teaspoon salt

1 teaspoon xanthan gum

½ cup (156 g) jam

1. Preheat the oven to 350°F (175°C).

2. Cream together the butter and sugar with a mixer on medium speed. Add the egg yolk and vanilla and mix to combine. In a separate bowl, whisk together the flour, salt, and xanthan gum; add to the butter-sugar mixture and mix to incorporate.

3. Shape the cookie dough into ½-tablespoon-size balls and place on an ungreased baking sheet 1 inch (2.5 cm) apart. Use your thumb or knuckle to make a deep indent in each cookie. (Make sure you don't go all the way through to the baking sheet.) Place ½ teaspoon of jam in each indent.

4. Bake for 12 to 15 minutes, until slightly golden on the edges. Allow to rest on the baking sheet for 5 minutes. Transfer to a wire rack to cool completely.

HIGH-ALTITUDE ADJUSTMENT: Increase the flour to 1¼ cups (156 g).

KIDS CAN . . .

* Collect ingredients from the pantry and refrigerator

* Measure ingredients

* Crack the egg and separate the yolk

* Dump ingredients into the mixing bowl

* Turn the mixer on/off

* Whisk the dry ingredients

* Scoop the dough and roll into balls

* Press in the center of the cookie with your thumb

* Fill the indented cookie with jam

To make this recipe . . . .

EGG-FREE

* In a small bowl, combine 1 teaspoon ground flaxseeds and 1 tablespoon water. Allow the mixture to set for at least 2 minutes and use in place of the egg yolk.

DAIRY/LACTOSE/CASEIN-FREE

* Substitute vegan shortening for the butter.

CORN-FREE

* Use arrowroot flour to make a corn-free version of the Artisan GF Flour Blend (page 26).

HONEY "GRAHAM" CRACKERS

• MAKES FORTY-TWO 2-INCH (5 CM) CRACKERS •

Graham crackers get their distinct flavor from wheat-based graham flour. Though there's no direct gluten-free equivalent, these honey "graham" crackers are pretty reminiscent. Pair them with chocolate and marshmallows roasted by an open fire to make s'mores, and you'll leave memories of the original graham crackers behind.

⅓ cup (77 g) packed brown sugar

2 cups (250 g) Artisan GF Flour Blend (page 27)

1 teaspoon xanthan gum

1 teaspoon GF baking powder

½ teaspoon baking soda

½ teaspoon salt

6 tablespoons (¾ stick, 84 g) butter, cut into pieces

¼ cup (85 g) honey

3 tablespoons milk

½ teaspoon GF pure vanilla extract

1. Preheat the oven to 350°F (175°C). Cut two pieces of parchment paper the size of your baking sheet.

2. Pulse the brown sugar, flour, xanthan gum, baking powder, baking soda, and salt in the food processor to combine. Add the butter and process until the butter is completely incorporated and the mixture looks like sand. Add the honey, milk, and vanilla and pulse until a dough forms and the mixture is uniformly mixed.

3. Place the dough on one piece of parchment and cover with the second piece. Roll the dough out to a rectangle that is about 12½ x 14½ inches (32 x 37 cm), about ⅛-inch (0.5 cm) thick. Remove the top piece of parchment paper.

4. Use a pizza cutter or knife to trim the edges to be completely straight and create a rectangle that is about 12 x 14 inches (30 x 36 cm). Cut the dough into 2-inch (5 cm) squares, but leave the entire sheet of dough in place on the parchment. Use a fork to poke holes in the dough.

5. Transfer the entire sheet of dough on the parchment onto the baking sheet. Bake for 20 minutes, until the crackers are just starting to brown on the edges.

6. Slide the piece of parchment paper off the baking sheet onto a wire rack and allow the crackers to cool completely. Break the crackers apart along the seams and store in an airtight container.

HIGH-ALTITUDE ADJUSTMENT: Increase the flour to 2½ cups (313 g).

KIDS CAN . . .

* Collect ingredients from the pantry and refrigerator

* Measure ingredients

* Dump ingredients into the food processor

* Press the food processor buttons

* Poke holes with a fork in the rolled-out dough

* Break the cooled graham cracker squares apart

To make this recipe . . . .

DAIRY/LACTOSE/CASEIN-FREE

* Substitute vegan shortening for the butter.
* Substitute nondairy milk for the cow's milk.

CORN-FREE

* Use arrowroot flour to make a corn-free version of the Artisan GF Flour Blend (page 26).
* Check the ingredients of your baking powder, which often contains cornstarch.

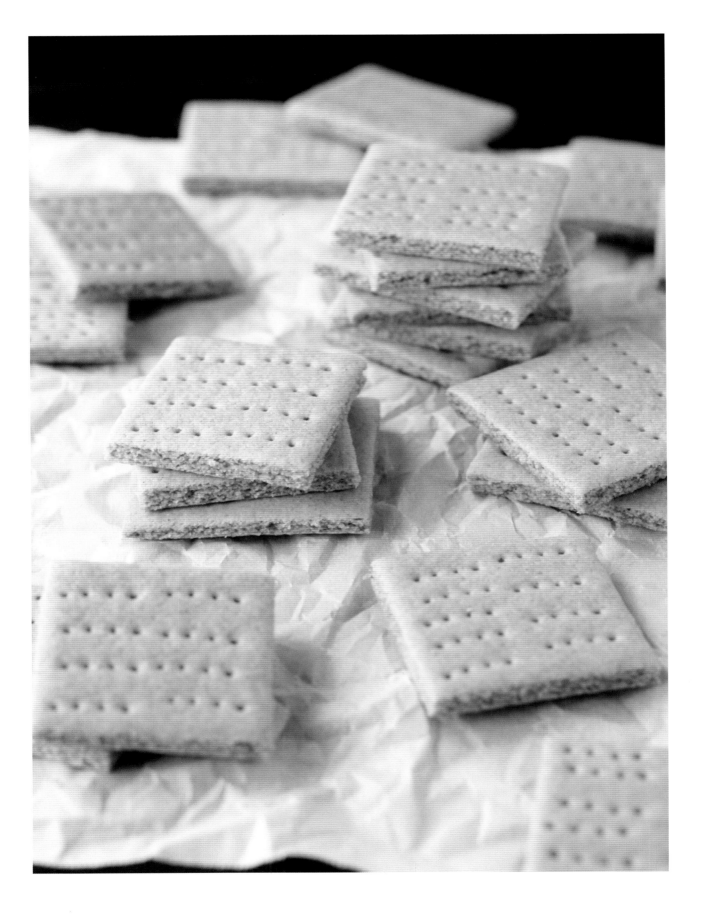

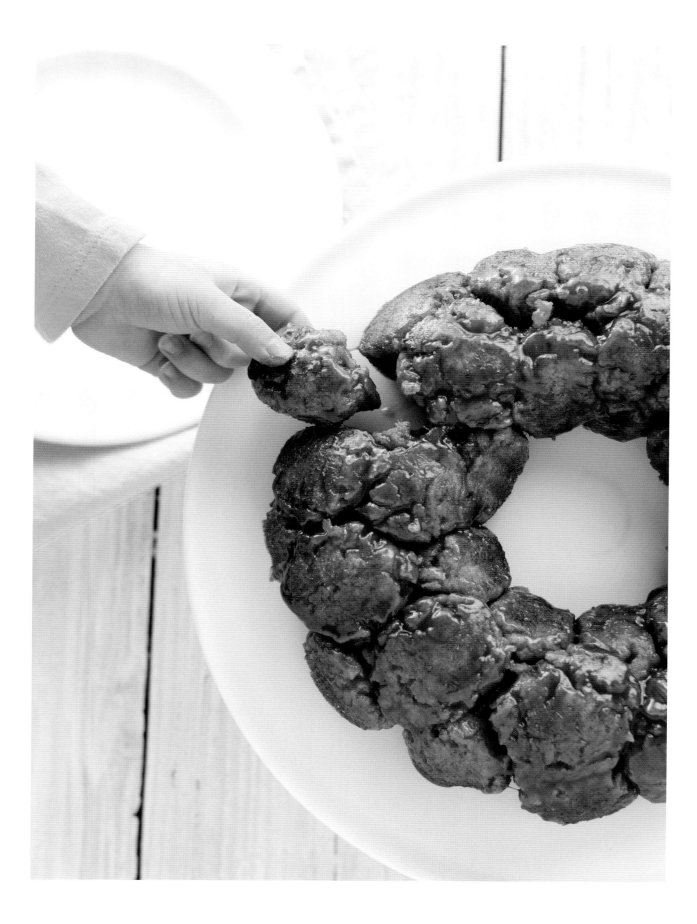

MONKEY BREAD

• MAKES 10 SERVINGS (1 BUNDT-CAKE-SIZE RING) •

Baked in a Bundt pan and made up of dozens of balls of fluffy dough that remind us of donut holes, this monkey bread makes for a gooey, sweet treat. Sticky fingers come with the territory!

DOUGH

6 tablespoons (90 ml) milk

¼ cup (54 g) plus 1 tablespoon granulated sugar

¼ cup (½ stick, 56 g) butter

¾ teaspoon salt

3 tablespoons warm water (about 115°F/45°C)

1 tablespoon yeast

2 eggs

2 cups (250 g) Artisan GF Flour Blend (page 27)

1 teaspoon xanthan gum

CINNAMON SUGAR

1 tablespoon ground cinnamon

¼ cup (54 g) sugar

1 tablespoon butter, melted

CARAMEL

¼ cup (½ stick, 56 g) butter

½ cup (115 g) packed brown sugar

2 tablespoons heavy cream

KIDS CAN . . .

* Collect ingredients from the pantry and refrigerator

* Measure ingredients

* Crack the eggs

* Dump ingredients into saucepan and mixing bowl

* Mix ingredients with a whisk or spoon

* Scoop the dough into balls

* Roll the dough in cinnamon sugar and place in pan

1. Grease a 10-inch (25 cm) Bundt pan with butter or nonstick cooking spray.

2. To make the dough, combine the milk, ¼ cup granulated sugar, butter, and salt in a small saucepan and heat until warm (about 115°F/45°C). Remove from the heat and allow the butter to continue to melt. Meanwhile, combine the warm water, yeast, and remaining 1 tablespoon sugar in a large bowl and let stand until mixture foams, about 5 minutes. Add the milk mixture and the eggs to the yeast mixture and whisk to combine. In a separate bowl, whisk together the flour and xanthan gum. Add to the yeast mixture and stir until smooth. The dough will be sticky. Set aside.

3. To make the cinnamon sugar, mix together the cinnamon and sugar in a shallow bowl and set aside with the melted butter in a small bowl nearby.

4. To make the caramel, heat the butter, brown sugar, and heavy cream in a saucepan over medium-high heat until the mixture comes to a boil, stirring occasionally. Boil for 30 seconds without stirring; remove from the heat.

5. To assemble the monkey bread, pour half of the caramel in the bottom of the prepared Bundt pan. Dip your fingers lightly in the melted butter and pinch off a scant-tablespoon-size piece of dough. Roll into a ball, roll in the cinnamon sugar to coat, and place in the Bundt pan. Repeat to create about 30 small balls in the bottom of the Bundt pan. Cover and place in a warm location and let rise for 1 hour, until the dough has doubled in size. Toward the end of the rise, preheat the oven to 350°F (175°C).

6. Gently rewarm the remaining caramel over low heat until it's pourable. Drizzle over the risen cinnamon sugar balls. Bake the monkey bread for 30 minutes. Let cool for 10 minutes. Flip out of the pan onto a plate and serve while warm.

(RECIPE CONTINUES)

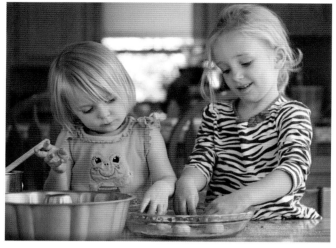
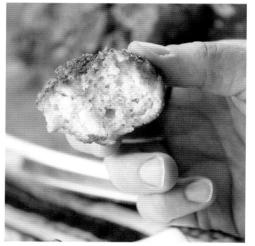
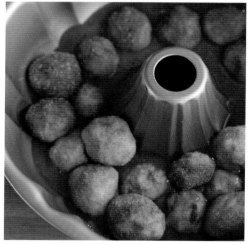
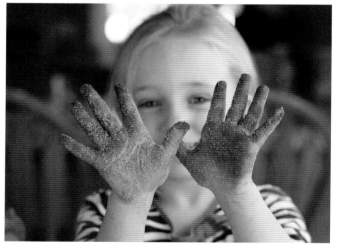

To make this recipe ....

EGG-FREE

- In a small bowl, combine 2 tablespoons ground flaxseeds and 6 tablespoons water. Allow the mixture to set for at least 2 minutes and use in place of the eggs in the dough.

DAIRY/LACTOSE/CASEIN-FREE

In the dough

- Substitute almond milk (or, for nut allergies, rice or hemp milk) for the cow's milk.
- Substitute melted coconut oil or melted vegan shortening for the butter.

In the cinnamon sugar

- Substitute melted coconut oil or melted vegan shortening for the butter.

In the caramel

- Substitute coconut oil for the butter.
- Substitute coconut cream for the heavy cream. (To make coconut cream, chill a can of full-fat coconut milk in the refrigerator overnight. Open the bottom of the can with a puncture can opener and pour the liquid off, reserving for another purpose, and just the cream will remain.)

CORN-FREE

- Use arrowroot flour to make a corn-free version of the Artisan GF Flour Blend (page 26).

CHOCOLATE BIRTHDAY CAKE WITH VANILLA FROSTING

• MAKES 12 TO 16 SERVINGS (ONE 8-INCH/20 CM TWO-LAYER CAKE OR ONE 13 X 9-INCH/33 X 23 CM CAKE) •

Every child deserves a great birthday cake; this moist chocolate cake really delivers.

CAKE

1 cup (2 sticks, 226 g) butter

1 cup (240 ml) water

½ cup (40 g) cocoa powder

2 cups (432 g) granulated sugar

2 eggs

1 cup (240 g) sour cream

1 teaspoon GF pure vanilla extract

2½ cups (313 g) Artisan GF Flour Blend (page 27)

2 teaspoons xanthan gum

1½ teaspoons GF baking powder

1½ teaspoons baking soda

½ teaspoon salt

FROSTING

1 cup (2 sticks, 226 g) butter, softened

4 cups (480 g) confectioners' sugar

¼ cup (60 ml) heavy cream

1 teaspoon GF pure vanilla extract

KIDS CAN . . .

* Collect ingredients from the pantry and refrigerator
* Measure ingredients
* Crack the eggs
* Dump ingredients into saucepan and mixing bowl
* Mix dry ingredients with a whisk
* Turn the mixer on/off
* Help frost the cake

1. Preheat the oven to 350°F (175°C). Grease two 8- or 9-inch (20 or 23 cm) cake pans (or one 13 x 9-inch/33 x 23 cm cake pan) with butter or nonstick cooking spray.* Line the bottom of the pans with parchment paper.

2. To make the cake, melt the butter in a saucepan over low heat. Add the water and cocoa and bring to a boil. Transfer to a large bowl and mix in the granulated sugar to dissolve the sugar and cool the mixture. When the mixture is lukewarm, mix in the eggs, sour cream, and vanilla to incorporate. Scrape down the sides of the bowl.

3. In a separate bowl, whisk together the flour, xanthan gum, baking powder, baking soda, and salt. Add to the cocoa mixture and mix for 10 seconds with a mixer on medium-low speed to incorporate. Scrape down the sides and mix for 5 seconds at high speed, just until smooth.

4. Divide the batter between the prepared pan(s). Gently tap the pan(s) on the countertop to release any air bubbles in the batter. Bake for 35 to 40 minutes, until a toothpick inserted in the center comes out clean. Cool fully in the pans.**

5. To make the frosting, cream all of the ingredients together until smooth, then mix on medium-high speed for about 3 minutes, until the frosting is very fluffy.

6. To assemble the layer cake, carefully flip out one layer from the pan and place on a cake plate. Remove the parchment paper. Spread about ¾ cup frosting on top of it. Place the second cake layer directly on top and remove the parchment paper. Cover the entire cake with the remaining frosting. (To make the single cake, flip out on a platter and frost the top and sides.)

(RECIPE CONTINUES)

*This recipe will also make 24 cupcakes. Bake for 25 minutes until a toothpick inserted in the center of a cupcake comes out clean.

**If making the recipe ahead, let the cake layers cool completely, then store in the freezer in separate zip-top bags or an airtight container, separated with parchment paper.

HIGH-ALTITUDE ADJUSTMENT: Increase the flour to 2¾ cups (344 g).

To make this recipe . . . .

EGG-FREE

- In a small bowl, combine 2 tablespoons ground flaxseeds and 6 tablespoons water. Allow the mixture to set for at least 2 minutes and use in place of the eggs in the cake batter.

DAIRY/LACTOSE/CASEIN-FREE

For the cake:
- Substitute vegan shortening for the butter.
- Substitute nondairy sour cream for the sour cream.

For the frosting:
- Substitute vegan shortening for the butter.
- Substitute coconut cream (see page 176) for the heavy cream.

CORN-FREE

- Use arrowroot flour to make a corn-free version of the Artisan GF Flour Blend (page 26).
- Check the ingredients of your baking powder, which often contains cornstarch.
- Use a corn-free confectioners' sugar, such as those made with tapioca, or make your own (see page 154).

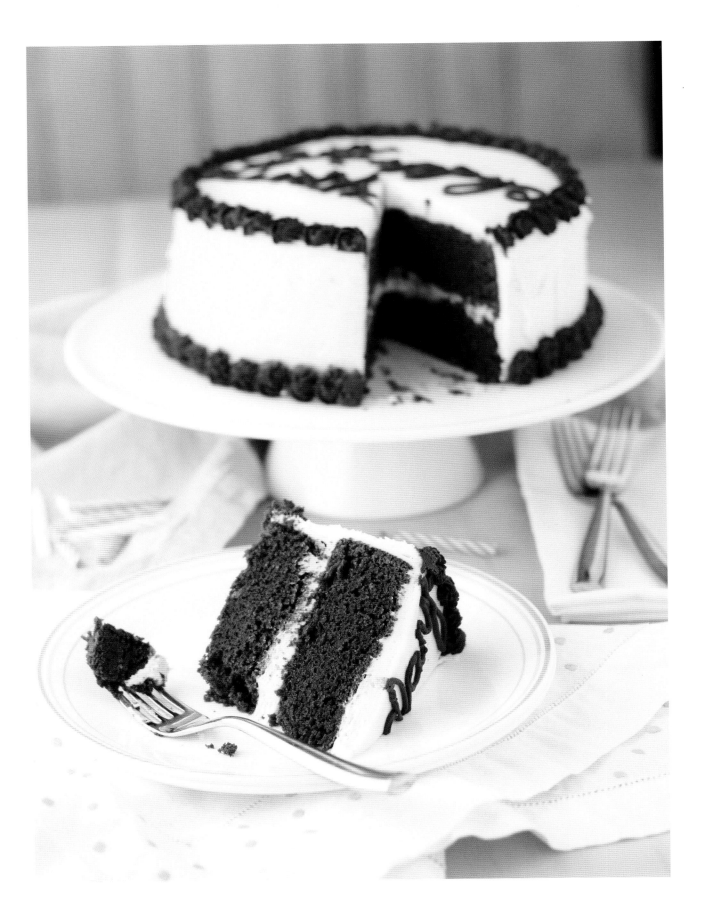

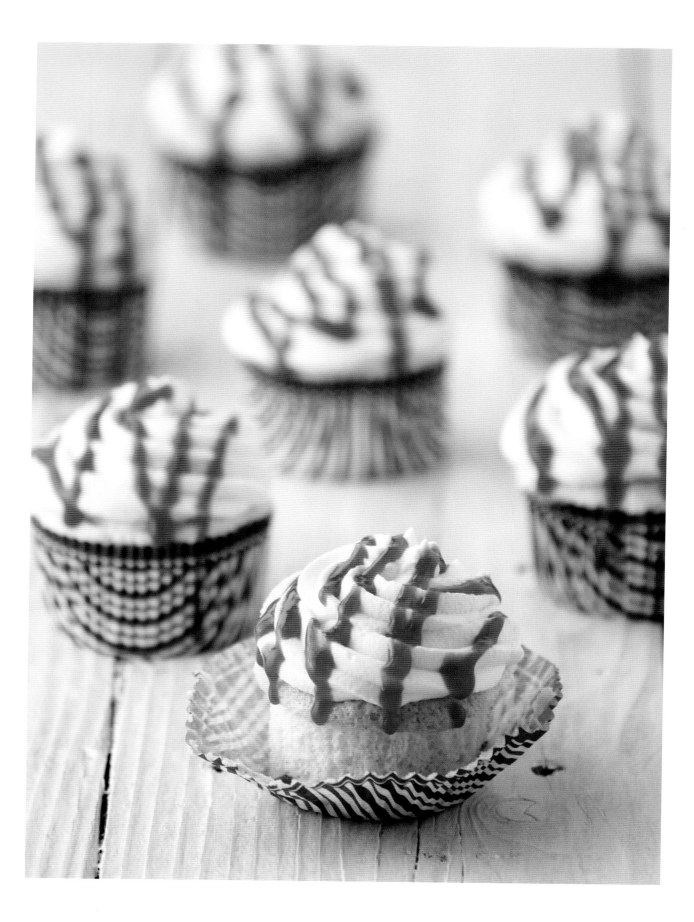

ANGEL FOOD CUPCAKES WITH RASPBERRY SAUCE AND WHIPPED CREAM

• MAKES 24 CUPCAKES •

These light and airy cupcakes, topped with whipped cream and bright red raspberry sauce, are already portioned for individual kid consumption.

CUPCAKES

1½ cups (355 ml) egg whites (from about 10 eggs), room temperature
2 teaspoons GF pure vanilla extract
½ teaspoon GF pure almond extract
1½ teaspoons cream of tartar
¼ teaspoon salt
½ cup (108 g) granulated sugar
1½ cups (180 g) sifted confectioners' sugar
1 cup (110 g) sifted Artisan GF Flour Blend (page 27)
1½ teaspoons xanthan gum

RASPBERRY SAUCE

⅓ cup (72 g) sugar
2 teaspoons cornstarch
¼ cup (60 ml) cold water
½ pint or 6 ounces (170 g) fresh or frozen raspberries

WHIPPED CREAM

1 cup (240 ml) heavy cream
1 tablespoon confectioners' sugar
1 teaspoon GF pure vanilla extract

KIDS CAN . . .

* Collect ingredients from the pantry and refrigerator
* Measure ingredients
* Crack the eggs and separate the egg whites
* Dump ingredients into mixing bowl
* Mix dry ingredients with a whisk
* Turn the mixer on/off
* Divide the batter between the muffin cups
* Decorate the cupcakes

1. Preheat the oven to 350°F (175°C). Line the cups of two 12-cup muffin tins with paper liners.

2. To make the cupcakes, whip the egg whites, vanilla extract, almond extract, cream of tartar, and salt with a mixer using the whisk attachment until soft peaks form. Add the granulated sugar a little at a time, beating until stiff peaks form. You want stiff peaks, but you do not want to overmix your egg whites or the cakes will deflate when they bake. Sift together the confectioners' sugar, flour, and xanthan gum. Carefully fold the flour mixture into the egg whites just until all the flour is mixed in.

3. Divide the batter among the 24 muffin cups and smooth the tops. Bake for 20 minutes, until the cupcakes are golden brown and the cracks on top of the cupcakes are dry. Remove from the muffin tins and cool completely on a wire rack.

4. Meanwhile, make the raspberry sauce: Combine the sugar and cornstarch in a saucepan. Stir in the water. Add the raspberries and bring to a boil. Simmer until clear and thickened, about 4 minutes. Strain through a fine-mesh strainer to remove seeds. Refrigerate until chilled.

5. To make the whipped cream, chill a metal bowl and whisk or beaters in the freezer for 5 minutes. Pour the cream into the cold bowl. Whip the cream until it starts to thicken. Add the confectioners' sugar and vanilla and whip until soft peaks form.

6. Frost the cooled cupcakes with the prepared whipped cream. Drizzle with the raspberry sauce (a spoon or piping bag with fine tip both work well).

To make this recipe . . . .

DAIRY/LACTOSE/CASEIN-FREE

• For the whipped cream, substitute the fluffy frosting from the Chocolate Cookies (page 163) or whipped coconut cream. To make whipped coconut cream: Chill a can of full-fat coconut milk in the refrigerator overnight. Open the bottom of the can with a puncture can opener and pour the liquid off (reserving for another purpose) and just the cream will remain. Place the coconut cream in a bowl and whip with a handheld mixer on medium-high speed until fluffy. Add the confectioners' sugar and vanilla extract called for in the recipe and whip until soft peaks form.

CORN-FREE

• Use arrowroot flour to make a corn-free version of the Artisan GF Flour Blend (page 26).
• Use a corn-free confectioners' sugar, such as those made with tapioca, or make your own (see page 154).
• Substitute tapioca starch for the cornstarch in the raspberry sauce.

APPLE CIDER DONUTS

· MAKES 12 DONUTS ·

Apple cider donuts remind us of the crisp days of fall and apple harvest season. We made these gluten-free donuts for a preschool trip to a local farm, and you couldn't tell the difference between them and the "real" thing!

2 cups (475 ml) apple cider

½ cup (108 g) sugar

¼ cup (½ stick, 56 g) butter, room temperature

2 eggs

½ cup (120 ml) buttermilk (see below to make your own)

2 teaspoons GF pure vanilla extract

2 cups (250 g) Artisan GF Flour Blend (page 27)

½ teaspoon xanthan gum

2 teaspoons GF baking powder

1 teaspoon baking soda

1 teaspoon ground cinnamon

¼ teaspoon ground nutmeg

½ teaspoon salt

CINNAMON SUGAR

¼ cup (54 g) sugar

1 tablespoon ground cinnamon

2 tablespoons butter, melted

KIDS CAN . . .

* Collect ingredients from the pantry and refrigerator

* Measure ingredients

* Crack the eggs

* Dump ingredients into mixing bowl

* Mix dry ingredients with a whisk

* Turn the mixer on/off

1. Bring the cider to a boil in a small saucepan and reduce to ½ cup (120 ml), about 20 minutes. Set aside.

2. Preheat the oven to 400°F (205°C). Grease a nonstick donut pan with nonstick cooking spray or butter.

3. Cream together the sugar and butter with a mixer on medium speed. Add the eggs and mix on low until incorporated. Mix in the reduced cider, buttermilk, and vanilla. In a separate bowl, whisk together the flour, xanthan gum, baking powder, baking soda, cinnamon, nutmeg, and salt; add to the cider mixture and mix until just smooth.

4. Use a pastry bag (or similar) with a ½-inch (1.25 cm) opening to pipe the dough into the greased donut pan cavities. Bake for 10 minutes, until the donuts spring back when touched. Remove from the pan and let cool on a wire rack. Repeat with the remaining dough to make 12 donuts total.

5. In a wide, shallow bowl, mix together the sugar and cinnamon. Brush an entire donut with melted butter and set the donut in the cinnamon sugar. Flip to coat the other side and sprinkle with cinnamon sugar to fill in any gaps. Repeat to coat all the donuts.

Make your own . . .

BUTTERMILK: Add 1½ teaspoons distilled white or apple cider vinegar to ½ cup milk. Let set for 5 minutes. This "acidified" buttermilk works well, though we prefer to use a true buttermilk. You can follow these same steps to make a nondairy buttermilk using almond, soy, or another nondairy milk.

To make this recipe . . . .

EGG-FREE

* In a small bowl, combine 2 tablespoons ground flaxseeds and 6 tablespoons water. Allow the mixture to set for at least 2 minutes and use in place of the eggs.

DAIRY/LACTOSE/CASEIN-FREE

* Make your own buttermilk (see above) with almond milk (or, for nut allergies, rice or hemp milk).
* Substitute melted coconut oil or melted vegan shortening for the butter.

CORN-FREE

* Use arrowroot flour to make a corn-free version of the Artisan GF Flour Blend (page 26).
* Check the ingredients of your baking powder, which often contains cornstarch.

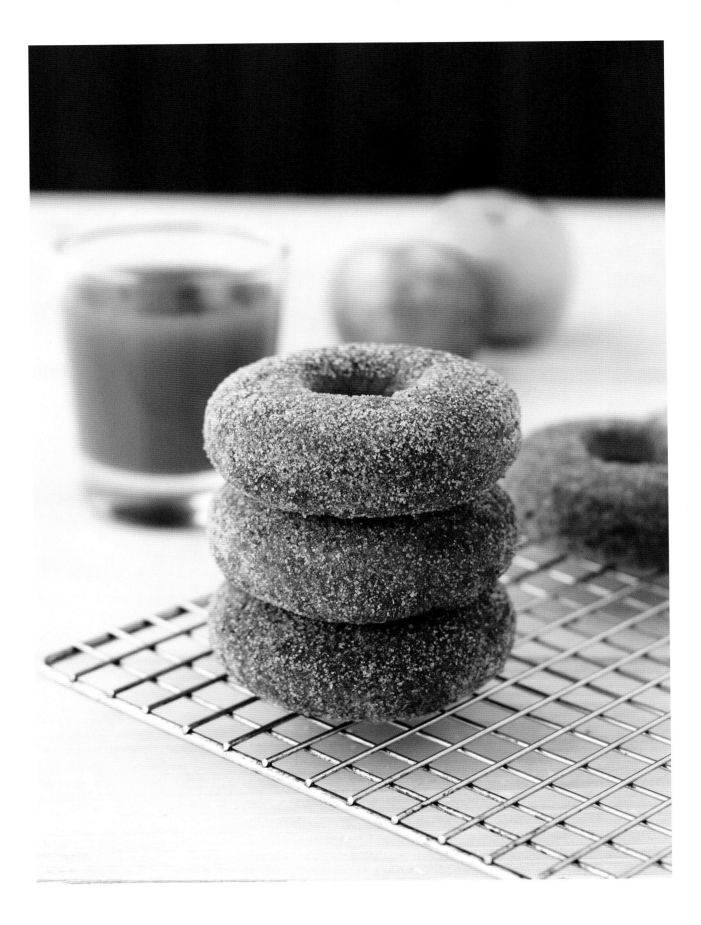

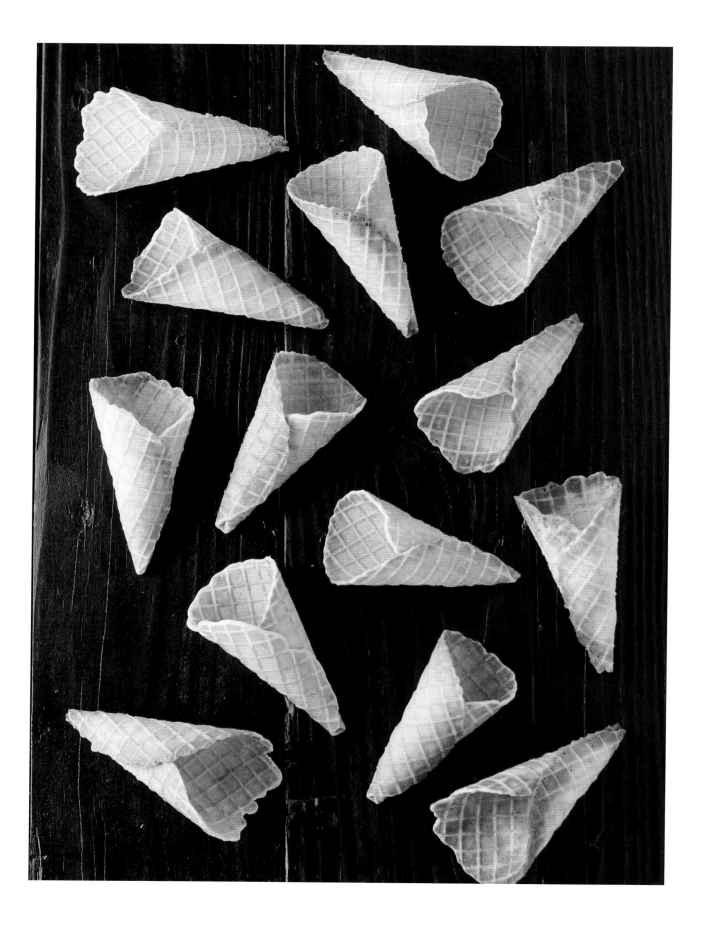

WAFFLE CONES

• MAKES 8 FULL-SIZE CONES OR 16 MINI CONES •

Gone are the days of you and your kids having to eat ice cream from a bowl with a spoon. These gluten-free waffle cones taste as good as the original.

2 eggs

½ cup (108 g) sugar

1 cup (125 g) Artisan GF Flour Blend (page 27)

¼ teaspoon salt

¼ cup (60 ml) milk

1 teaspoon GF pure vanilla extract

¼ cup (½ stick, 56 g) butter, melted

KIDS CAN . . .

* Collect ingredients from the pantry and refrigerator
* Measure ingredients
* Crack the eggs
* Dump ingredients into mixing bowl
* Mix ingredients with a whisk
* Scoop batter onto the griddle

1. Preheat a waffle cone maker to level 4 (medium-high). If you don't have a waffle cone maker, you could also use a panini or pizzelle press.

2. In a large bowl, whisk together the eggs and sugar until the eggs lighten in color. Add the flour and salt and whisk until the mixture is smooth. Add the milk and vanilla and whisk until smooth. Add the melted butter and whisk again until completely incorporated.

3. Using a cookie scoop or spoon, place 1 tablespoon for a small cone or 2 tablespoons for a standard-size cone on the center of the waffle cone maker. Close the lid and cook for 1 minute. Check to see if the cone is dark enough and cook for up to 30 seconds more.

4. Remove the cone from the maker and place on a clean towel. Using a conical waffle cone roller (or a piece of sturdy cardstock or paperboard, such as a cereal box, formed into a cone) carefully roll the cone around the roller, ensuring the bottom is closed so ice cream does not sneak out.* Hold the rolled cone in place on the mold for 10 seconds and set aside.

5. Repeat with the remaining batter.

*If you do have a small opening at the bottom of the cone, place a chocolate chip or two inside to prevent the ice cream from running out the bottom.

To make this recipe . . . .

EGG-FREE

* In a small bowl, combine 2 tablespoons ground flaxseeds and 6 tablespoons water. Allow the mixture to set for at least 2 minutes and use in place of the eggs.

DAIRY/LACTOSE/CASEIN-FREE

* Substitute almond milk (or, for nut allergies, rice or hemp milk) for the cow's milk.
* Substitute melted vegan shortening for the butter.

CORN-FREE

* Use arrowroot flour to make a corn-free version of the Artisan GF Flour Blend (page 26).

ICE CREAM SANDWICHES

• MAKES 12 SANDWICHES •

When summer rolls around, it's time to break out the ice cream sandwiches. The chocolate "cake-cookie" is just the right taste and texture to recreate this classic.

¾ cup (162 g) sugar

¼ cup plus 2 tablespoons (30 g) cocoa powder

¾ cup (1½ sticks, 170 g) butter, melted

2 eggs

1½ teaspoons GF pure vanilla extract

¾ cup (94 g) Artisan GF Flour Blend (page 27)

¾ teaspoon xanthan gum

¼ teaspoon salt

4 cups (648 g) ice cream

KIDS CAN . . .

* Collect ingredients from the pantry and refrigerator

* Measure ingredients

* Crack the eggs

* Dump ingredients into mixing bowl

* Mix ingredients with a whisk or spoon

* Help spread ice cream

1. Preheat the oven to 350°F (175°C). Spray a half sheet pan or rimmed baking sheet (about 11 x 16 inches/28 x 41 cm) with nonstick cooking spray and line with parchment paper. (The spray will keep the parchment from sliding around).

2. In a medium bowl, mix together the sugar, cocoa powder, and melted butter. Add the eggs and vanilla (make sure the butter mixture is not too hot as you do not want to cook your eggs), and stir until smooth. In a separate bowl, whisk together the flour, xanthan gum, and salt; add to the cocoa mixture and stir to incorporate.

3. Spread the batter on the parchment paper, going all the way to the edge of the pan; using an offset spatula helps with this process. You want to spread the batter as evenly as you can; it will not spread much while it bakes. Bake for 10 minutes. Allow to cool completely on the baking sheet.

4. While the cake is cooling, pull the ice cream out of the freezer to soften a little bit (you do not want it too soft as it will become oozy and seep out of the sandwich while it freezes, but a little softening helps to spread it).

5. Slide the cake with the parchment off the pan. Cut it in half cross-wise to make two equal rectangles. Slide one half, top-side down, onto the middle of two overlapping pieces of plastic wrap that are about 2 feet (60 cm) long. Spread the ice cream on the top of the cake. Top with the remaining cake half, top-side up. Wrap with plastic wrap and freeze for at least 4 hours.

6. Trim the edges of the large rectangle to make the edges completely straight. Make 3 lengthwise cuts and 2 cross-wise cuts to create 12 rectangles about 2 x 4 inches (5 x 10 cm).

To make this recipe . . . .

DAIRY/LACTOSE/CASEIN-FREE
* Substitute melted vegan shortening for the butter.
* Substitute nondairy ice cream for the ice cream.

CORN-FREE
* Use arrowroot flour to make a corn-free version of the Artisan GF Flour Blend (page 26).
* Check the ingredients of your ice cream, which often contains corn syrup or similar.

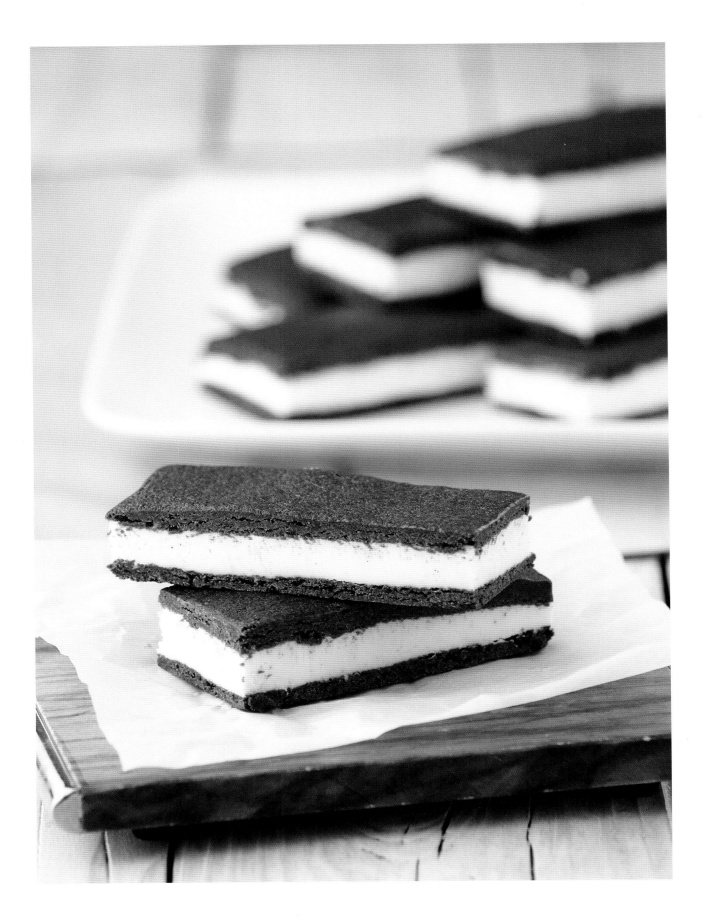

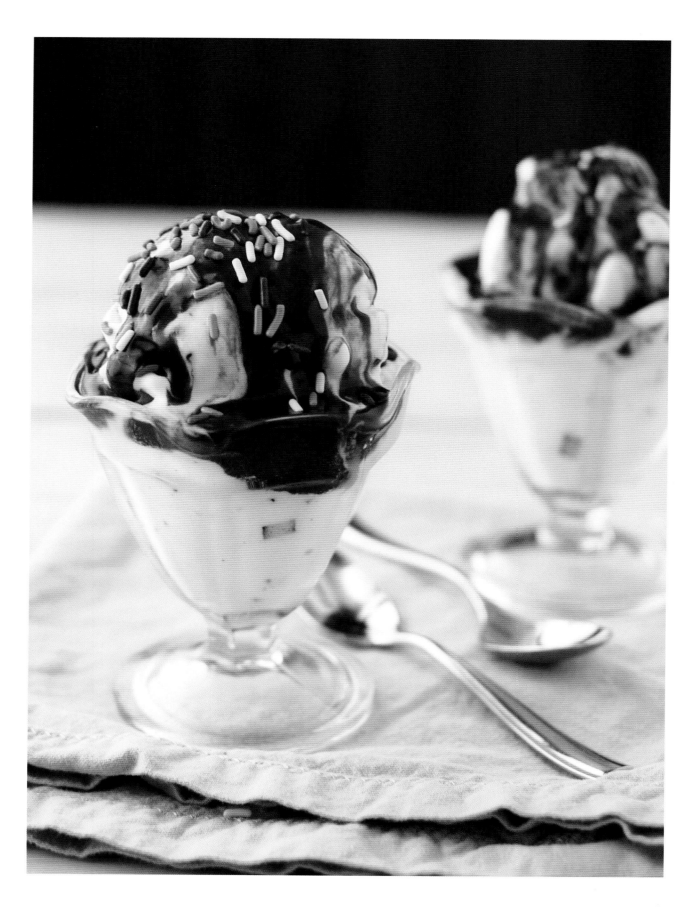

CHOCOLATE HOT FUDGE SAUCE

• MAKES 1½ CUPS •

What do you get when you mix the taste of rich hot fudge with the pourable consistency of chocolate sauce? This recipe! Plus, it's free of the corn syrup so common in other similar sauces.

½ cup (108 g) sugar

¼ cup (20 g) cocoa powder

½ cup (166 g) agave nectar

½ cup (120 ml) half-and-half

3 tablespoons butter

¼ teaspoon salt

¼ teaspoon GF pure vanilla extract

1. In a medium saucepan, whisk together the sugar and cocoa powder. Add the agave nectar, half-and-half, butter, and salt.

2. Bring to a boil over medium heat, stirring. Boil for 5 minutes, stirring continuously.

3. Remove from the heat and stir in the vanilla extract.

4. Serve when warm, not hot, or store in the refrigerator for up to 1 month.

KIDS CAN . . .

✳ Collect ingredients from the pantry and refrigerator

✳ Measure ingredients

✳ Add ingredients to the saucepan

✳ Stir the sauce while cooking

To make this recipe . . . .

DAIRY/LACTOSE/CASEIN-FREE AND VEGAN

● Substitute coconut milk for the half-and-half and coconut oil for the butter.

REFINED-SUGAR-FREE

● Substitute coconut sugar for the granulated sugar.

RICE PUDDING

This refined-sugar-free rice pudding—with just the right amount of cinnamon and nutmeg—is rich and creamy. At the ripe old age of two-and-a-half, our daughter Charlotte confidently rejected a popular store-bought brand of rice pudding in favor of our homemade version.

6 cups (1.4 liters) milk

1 cup (190 g) long-grain white rice

½ teaspoon salt

1 cup (240 ml) half-and-half

⅔ cup (160 ml) agave nectar

3 eggs

2 teaspoons GF pure vanilla extract

1 teaspoon ground cinnamon

¼ teaspoon ground nutmeg

Boiling water

KIDS CAN . . .

＊ Collect ingredients from the pantry and refrigerator

＊ Measure ingredients

＊ Crack the eggs

＊ Dump ingredients into saucepan and mixing bowl

＊ Mix ingredients with a whisk or spoon

1. In a large saucepan, combine the milk, rice, and salt and bring to a simmer over medium-high heat, stirring frequently to prevent sticking on the bottom. Turn the heat down to medium and simmer uncovered for 30 minutes, until the rice is soft and the mixture is very thick.

2. Preheat the oven to 350°F (175°C). Grease a 9 x 9-inch (23 x 23 cm) baking dish with nonstick cooking spray.

3. In a bowl, whisk together the half-and-half, agave nectar, eggs, vanilla, cinnamon, and nutmeg. Slowly add the cooked rice to the milk mixture and whisk until completely incorporated.

4. Pour the mixture into the prepared pan. Place the pan in a larger baking pan and set on a rack in the preheated oven. Pour boiling water in the larger pan to come halfway up the sides of the baking dish. Bake for 40 to 45 minutes, until the pudding is just set at the edges when the pan is jiggled. Remove from the hot water bath, cool, and enjoy! Store in an airtight container in the refrigerator for up to 5 days.

ALTERNATE METHOD: To save prep time, mix the uncooked rice with all of the other ingredients in a large bowl and pour into the greased baking pan. Bake in the oven in the water bath for 70 to 90 minutes, until the pudding is set around the edges. The result will be not quite as thick and creamy, but still delicious.

To make this recipe . . . .

DAIRY/LACTOSE/CASEIN-FREE

● Substitute 3½ cups (830 ml) water and one 13.5-ounce (400 ml) can coconut milk for the 6 cups of milk in step 1, and substitute a second can of coconut milk for the 1 cup half-and-half.

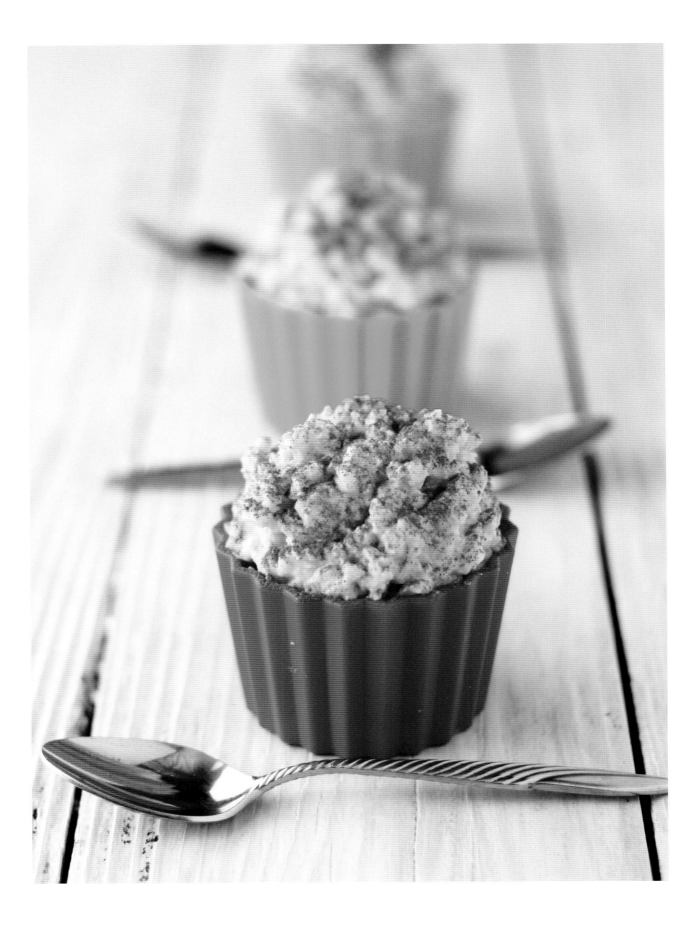

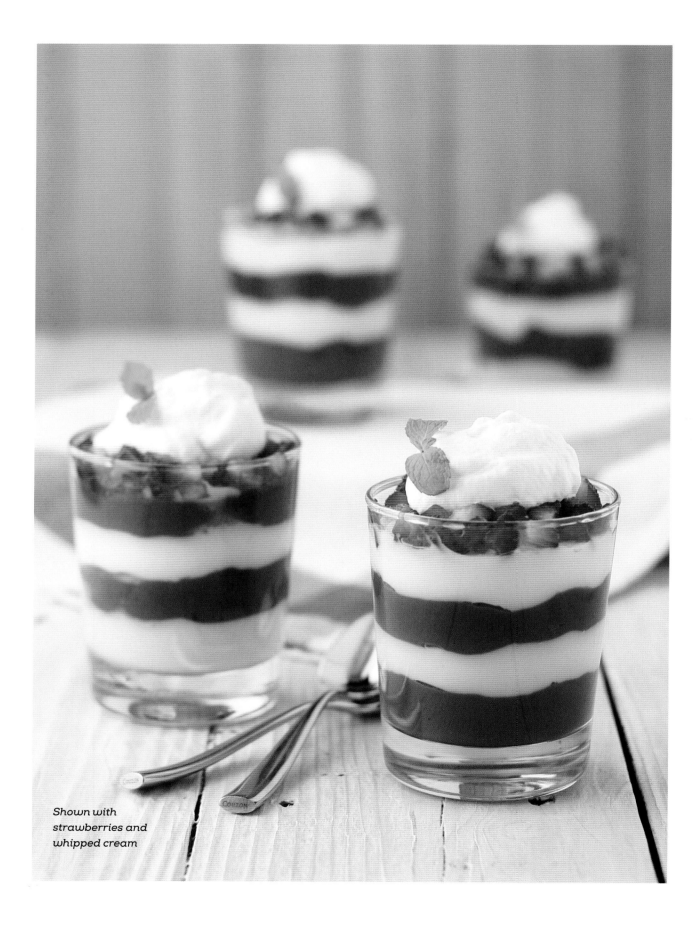

Shown with strawberries and whipped cream

VANILLA AND CHOCOLATE PUDDING

• MAKES 2 CUPS (4 SERVINGS) OF EACH FLAVOR •

These silky smooth puddings are the best of two worlds: simple and delicious. They're great on their own, layered and topped with fresh fruit such as diced strawberries, or frozen to make pudding pops.

VANILLA PUDDING

2 cups (475 ml) milk

¼ cup (54 g) sugar

3 tablespoons cornstarch

2 egg yolks

1 tablespoon butter

1 teaspoon GF pure vanilla extract

CHOCOLATE PUDDING

2 cups (475 ml) milk

⅓ cup (72 g) sugar

3 tablespoons cornstarch

2 egg yolks

1 tablespoon butter

1 teaspoon GF pure vanilla extract

2 ounces (57 g) unsweetened chocolate, pieces or chopped

1. To make the vanilla and/or chocolate pudding, in a saucepan, whisk together the milk, sugar, cornstarch, and egg yolks, until the cornstarch is completely dissolved. Bring the mixture to a boil over medium-high heat, whisking constantly. Boil for 1 minute, continuing to whisk. Remove from the heat and whisk in the butter and vanilla. If making chocolate pudding, whisk in the chocolate until melted.

2. Pour into 4 serving bowls or cups, cover, and refrigerate to cool and set.

3. You can also pour the warm pudding into pop molds and freeze to make pudding pops. (Each batch of vanilla or chocolate pudding makes five ⅓-cup pops.)

KIDS CAN . . .

* Collect ingredients from the pantry and refrigerator

* Measure ingredients

* Crack eggs and separate the egg yolks

* Dump ingredients into saucepan

* Mix ingredients with a whisk

To make this recipe . . . .

SOY-FREE
- Confirm that your chocolate does not contain soy lecithin.

DAIRY/LACTOSE/CASEIN-FREE
- Substitute almond milk or coconut milk (or, for nut allergies, rice or hemp milk) for the cow's milk.
- Omit the butter.

CORN-FREE
- Substitute tapioca starch for the cornstarch.

REFINED-SUGAR-FREE
- Substitute 3 tablespoons agave nectar for the sugar in the vanilla pudding, ¼ cup agave nectar for the sugar in the chocolate pudding.

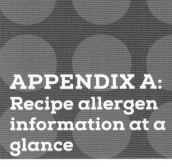

	GLUTEN/WHEAT-FREE	PEANUT-FREE	TREE-NUT-FREE	SOY-FREE	FISH-FREE	SHELLFISH-FREE	EGG-FREE	DAIRY/LACTOSE/CASEIN-FREE	CORN-FREE	REFINED-SUGAR-FREE	VEGETARIAN	VEGAN	GRAIN-FREE
BREAKFASTS													
Traditional Pancakes (page 31)	S	S	S	S	S	S	I	I	I	S	S	I	
Sweet Potato Pancakes (page 32)	S	S	S	S	S	S	I	I	I	S	S	I	
French Toast Sticks (page 35)	S	S	S	S	S	S		I	I	I	S		
Hot Cereal (page 36)	S	S	I	S	S	S	S	I	S	I	S	I	
Blueberry Mini Muffins (page 39)	S	S	S	S	S	S	I	I	I		S	I	
Banana Mini Muffins (page 40)	S	S	S	S	S	S	I	S	I	S	S	I	
Zucchini Bread (page 43)	S	S	S	S	S	S	I	S	I		S	I	
Scones (page 44)	S	S	S	S	S	S	I	I	I	I	S	I	
Cinnamon Granola Bars (page 47)	S	S	I	S	S	S	S	I	S	S	S	S	
Hash Brown Patties (page 48)	S	S	S	S	S	S	S	S	S	S	S	S	S
Scrambled Omelet (page 51)	S	S	S	S	S	S		I	S	S	I		S
Personal Quiches (page 52)	S	S	S	S	S	S		I	I	S	I		
Rainbow of Smoothies (page 55)	S	S	I	S	S	S	S	S	S	S	S	S	S
SIDES AND SNACKS													
Fruit Strips (page 59)	S	S	S	S	S	S	S	S	S	I	S	I	S
Fruit Kabobs with Yogurt Fondue (page 60)	S	S	S	S	S	S	S		S	S	S		S
Fruit Salsa with Cinnamon Chips (page 63)	S	S	S	S	S	S	S	I	I	I	S	I	
Cinnamon Apples (page 64)	S	S	S	S	S	S	S	I	S	S	S	I	S
Caprese Pops (page 67)	S	S	S	S	S	S	S		S	S	S		S
Hummus (page 68)	S	S	S	S	S	S	S	S	S	S	S	S	S

S = Standard recipe is suitable as written
I = Either confirm the status of an ingredient or follow instructions for a substitution

	GLUTEN/WHEAT-FREE	PEANUT-FREE	TREE-NUT-FREE	SOY-FREE	FISH-FREE	SHELLFISH-FREE	EGG-FREE	DAIRY/LACTOSE/CASEIN-FREE	CORN-FREE	REFINED-SUGAR-FREE	VEGETARIAN	VEGAN	GRAIN-FREE
Kale Chips (page 71)	S	S	S	S	S	S	S	S	S	S	S	S	S
Brussels Bites (page 72)	S	S	S	S	S	S	S	S	S	S	S	S	S
Breaded Zucchini Chips (page 75)	S	S	S	S	S	S	I	I	I	I	S	I	
Sweet Potater Tots (page 76)	S	S	S	S	S	S	S	S	I	S	S	S	I
Cashew Coconut Chia Bars (page 79)	S	S		S	S	S	S	S	S	S	S	S	S
Sandwich Bread (page 80)	S	S	S	S	S	S	I	I	I	I	S	I	
Dinner Rolls (page 83)	S	S	S	S	S	S	I	I	I	I	S	I	
Tofu Popcorn (page 85)	S	S	S		S	S	S	S	I	S	S	S	I
Soft Pretzels (page 87)	S	S	S	S	S	S	I	I	I	I	S	I	
MAIN MEALS													
Pesto Mac and Cheese (page 91)	S	S	I	S	S	S	I	I	I	S	S	I	
Spaghetti Squash "Pasta" with Easy Marinara Sauce (page 92)	S	S	S	S	S	S	S	S	S	S	S	S	S
Pumpkin Gnocchi Nuggets (page 95)	S	S	S	S	S	S		I	I	S	S		
Personal Pizzas (page 96)	S	S	S	S	S	S	S	I	I	I	I	I	
Lentil Salad (page 99)	S	S	S	S	S	S	S	I	S	S	S	I	S
Asian Quinoa Salad (page 100)	S	S	S	I	S	S	S	S	S	S	S	I	
Corn Chowder (page 103)	S	S	S	S	S	S	S	I		S	I	I	
Jumbo Pigs in a Blanket (page 104)	S	S	S	S	S	S	S	S	I		S	I	I
Quesadillas (page 107)	S	S	S	S	S	S	S	I	I		S	I	
Pupusa Pockets (page 108)	S	S	S	S	S	S	S	I			S	S	I
Grilled Cheese (page 111)	S	S	S	S	S	S	S	I	I		S	S	I
Tortilla Sandwich Wraps (page 112)	S	S	S	S	S	S	S	S	I		S	S	S
Spanakopita Hand Pies (page 115)	S	S	S	S	S	S	I		I		S	S	
Fish Sticks (page 117)	S	S	S	S		S	I	I	I	I			
Coconut Shrimp with Mango Dipping Sauce (page 121)	S	S	I	S	S			S	S	I			
Chicken Fried Rice (page 123)	S	S	S	I	S	S	I	S	S	S	I		
Chicken and Broccoli Asian Noodle Bowl (page 124)	S	S	S	I	I	S	S	S	I	I	I	I	
Slow Cooker Chicken Noodle Soup (page 127)	S	S	S	S	S	S	S	S	I	S			
Chicken Fingers (page 128)	S	S	S	S	S	S	I	I	I	I			
Mediterranean Chicken Skewers (page 131)	S	S	S	S	S	S	S	I	S	S	I	I	S

	GLUTEN/WHEAT-FREE	PEANUT-FREE	TREE-NUT-FREE	SOY-FREE	FISH-FREE	SHELLFISH-FREE	EGG-FREE	DAIRY/LACTOSE/CASEIN-FREE	CORN-FREE	REFINED-SUGAR-FREE	VEGETARIAN	VEGAN	GRAIN-FREE
Teriyaki Chicken (page 132)	S	S	S	I	S	S	S	S	S		I	I	S
Cornbread Taco Muffins (page 135)	S	S	S	S	S	S		I		S			
Italian Meatball Subs (page 137)	S	S	S	S	S	S		I	I	I			
Turkey Burgers on Potato Rolls (page 139)	S	S	S	S	S	S	I	I	I	I			
Quinoa Meatloaf (page 142)	S	S	S	S	I	S	I	I	S	S			
Slow Cooker Green Chili with Pork (page 145)	S	S	S	S	S	S	S	I	S	S			
Spaghetti Bolognese (page 146)	S	S	S	S	S	S	S	S	I	S			
Beef Stroganoff (page 149)	S	S	S	S	S	S	S	I	I	S			
TASTY TREATS													
Frozen Fruit Pops (page 153)	S	S	S	S	S	S	S	S	S	S	S	S	S
Lemon Bars (page 154)	S	S		S	S	S		I	I		S		
Chocolate Peanut Butter Brownies (page 157)	S	I	S	I	S	S	I	I	I		S		
Fig Einsteins (page 159)	S	S	S	S	S	S	I	I	I		S		
Chocolate Cookies with Fluffy Frosting (page 163)	S	S	S	S	S	S		I	I		S		
Peanut Butter Cookies with Chocolate Clovers (page 164)	S	I	S	I	S	S	I	I	I		S		
Snickerdoodles (page 167)	S	S	S	S	S	S	I	I	I		S		
Chocolate Chip Cookies (page 168)	S	S	S	I	S	S	I	I	I		S		
Thumbprint Jam Cookies (page 171)	S	S	S	S	S	S	I	I	I		S		
Honey "Graham" Crackers (page 172)	S	S	S	S	S	S	S	I	I		S		
Monkey Bread (page 175)	S	S	S	S	S	S	I	I	I		S		
Chocolate Birthday Cake with Vanilla Frosting (page 177)	S	S	S	S	S	S	I	I	I		S		
Angel Food Cupcakes with Raspberry Sauce and Whipped Cream (page 181)	S	S	S	S	S	S		I	I		S		
Apple Cider Donuts (page 182)	S	S	S	S	S	S	I	I	I		S		
Waffle Cones (page 185)	S	S	S	S	S	S	I	I	I		S		
Ice Cream Sandwiches (page 186)	S	S	S	S	S	S		I	I		S		
Chocolate Hot Fudge Sauce (page 189)	S	S	S	S	S	S	S	I	S	I	S	I	S
Rice Pudding (page 190)	S	S	S	S	S	S		I	S	S	S		
Vanilla and Chocolate Pudding (page 193)	S	S	S	S	S	S		I	I	I	S		

S = Standard recipe is suitable as written
I = Either confirm the status of an ingredient or follow instructions for a substitution

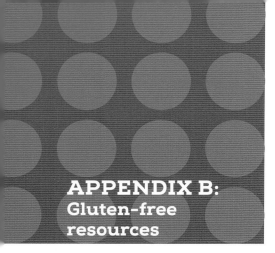

APPENDIX B:
Gluten-free resources

Medical information

There are many local sources of information about gluten-related issues. Here we list only the most prominent, nationally recognized research centers and other medical resources.

Celiac Center, Harvard Medical School/Beth Israel Deaconess Medical Center
    bidmc.org/celiaccenter

Celiac Disease, Mayo Clinic
    mayoclinic.com/health/celiac-disease/DS00319

Celiac Disease and Gluten Sensitivity Center, Stony Brook Children's Hospital
    stonybrookchildrens.org/specialties-services/clinical-programs/celiac-gluten

Celiac Disease Awareness Campaign, National Institutes of Health
    celiac.nih.gov
    digestive.niddk.nih.gov/ddiseases/pubs/celiac

Celiac Disease Center, Columbia University Medical Center
    celiacdiseasecenter.org

Celiac Disease Center, University of Chicago
    cureceliacdisease.org

Center for Celiac Research & Treatment, MassGeneral Hospital for Children (formerly associated with the University of Maryland Medical Center)
    celiaccenter.org

Kogan Celiac Center of Barnabas Health
    http://www.barnabashealth.org/Ambulatory-Care/Our-Services/Celiac-Disease-Center.aspx

Support and advocacy organizations

American Celiac Disease Alliance
americanceliac.org

Celiac Disease Foundation
celiac.org

Celiac Support Association
csaceliacs.info

Food Allergy Research & Education
foodallergy.org

Gluten Intolerance Group
gluten.net

National Foundation for Celiac Awareness
celiaccentral.org

Resources for gluten-free families and children

Kids Central, National Foundation for Celiac Awareness
Includes a Kids Page with games, recipes, encouraging "pep talks" (including one from Pete!), and more. Also includes a Parents Page with medical information, a back to school guide, and gluten-free-friendly summer camps for kids and teens.
celiaccentral.org/kids

R.O.C.K.—Raising Our Celiac Kids
A nationwide network of support groups for gluten-free kids and their parents.
celiackids.com

Certification and labeling standards

Codex Alimentarius
www.codexalimentarius.org

Food Allergen Labeling and Consumer Protection Act of 2004, US Food and Drug Administration
tinyurl.com/USFDAFALCPA2004

Gluten-Free Certification Organization, Gluten Intolerance Group
gfco.org

Gluten-Free Certification Program, National Foundation for Celiac Awareness/Canadian Celiac Association
gf-cert.org

Gluten-Free Labeling of Foods, US Food and Drug Administration
tinyurl.com/USFDAGlutenFreeRuling

Magazines

Allergic Living
    allergicliving.com

Delight Gluten Free Magazine
    delightglutenfree.com

Gluten-Free Living
    glutenfreeliving.com

Living Without
    livingwithout.com

Simply Gluten Free Magazine
    simplyglutenfreemag.com

Blogs

There are literally hundreds of gluten-free blogs today. This list is just the very tip of the iceberg. But we've chosen here all blogs that are gluten-free (of course), written by parents, and which cover a range of gluten-free perspectives: straight up GF, GF and Paleo, GF and dairy-free, GF and refined-sugar-free, and GF and Top 8 allergen-free.

A Girl Defloured
    agirldefloured.com

Cybele Pascal, The Allergy-Friendly Cook
    cybelepascal.com

Elana's Pantry
    elanaspantry.com

Gluten Free Easily
    glutenfreeeasily.com

Gluten-Free Girl
    glutenfreegirl.com

Silvana's Kitchen
    silvanaskitchen.com

Simply Sugar & Gluten-Free
    simplysugarandglutenfree.com

The Spunky Coconut
    www.thespunkycoconut.com

The Whole Gang
    thewholegang.org

NOTES

1   "Prevalence of Celiac Disease in At-Risk and Not-At-Risk Groups in the United States." *Archives of Internal Medicine.* February 2003, 163: 286–292.

2   "Assessing Causality and Persistence in Associations Between Family Dinners and Adolescent Wellbeing." University of California—Los Angeles, California Center for Population Research. Accessed August 2013. http://papers.ccpr.ucla.edu/papers/PWP-CCPR-2011-003/PWP-CCPR-2011-003.pdf
    "Development of eating behaviors among children and adolescents." *Pediatrics.* March 1998, 101(3 pt 2): 539–549.
    "Evaluation of a cooking skills programme in parents of young children—a longitudinal study." *Public Health Nutrition.* February 2013, 12: 1–9.
    "Family Nutrition: The Truth About Family Meals." University of Florida IFAS Extension. Accessed August 2013. http://edis.ifas.ufl.edu/fy1061
    "Influence of parental attitudes in the development of children eating behaviour." *British Journal of Nutrition.* February 1993, 99(suppl 1): S22–S25.
    "Is Frequency of Shared Family Meals Related to the Nutritional Health of Children and Adolescents?" *Pediatrics.* June 2011, 127(6): e1565–e1574.
    "Kids Who Cook Hungrier for Healthy Food Choices." University of Alberta. Accessed August 2013. http://www.news.ualberta.ca/newsarticles/2012/06/kidswhocookhungrierforhealthyfoodchoices
    "Overcoming picky eating. Eating enjoyment as a central aspect of children's eating behaviors." *Appetite.* April 2012, 58(2): 567–574.
    "Parenting in Context: Do Family Meals Really Make a Difference?" Cornell Univesity, College of Human Ecology. Accessed August 2013. http://www.human.cornell.edu/pam/outreach/parenting/research/upload/Family-Meal-times-2.pdf
    "Why Mealtime Matters." *The Power of Family Meals.* Accessed August 2013. http://poweroffamilymeals.com/resources/about

3   "Supermarket Facts: Industry Overview 2011–2012." Food Marketing Institute. Accessed August 2013. http://www.fmi.org/research-resources/supermarket-facts

4   "Gluten-free foods industry worth $4.2 billion." *Fox News.* October 23, 2012. Accessed August 2013. http://www.foxnews.com/health/2012/10/23/gluten-free-foods-industry-worth-42-billion/

5   "Gluten-Fee Is Still Going Gangbusters." Packaged Facts. October 19, 2012. Accessed August 2013. http://www.packagedfacts.com/about/release.asp?id=3033

6   "Gluten-free Foods—US—January 2012." Mintel. Accessed August 2013. http://oxygen.mintel.com/sinatra/oxygen/list/id=590142&type=RCItem#0_1____page_RCItem=0

7   "Food Allergies: What You Need To Know." U.S. Food and Drug Administration. April 17, 2013. Accessed August 2013. http://www.fda.gov/Food/ResourcesForYou/Consumers/ucm079311.htm

8   "Guidance for Industry: Questions and Answers Regarding Food Allergens." U.S. Food and Drug Administration. October 2006. Updated February 28, 2013. Accessed August 2013. http://www.fda.gov/Food/GuidanceRegulation/GuidanceDocumentsRegulatoryInformation/Allergens/ucm059116.htm

9   "What is Gluten-Free? FDA Has an Answer." U.S. Food and Drug Administration. August 2, 2013. Accessed August 2013. http://www.fda.gov/ForConsumers/ConsumerUpdates/ucm363069.htm

10 "Codex Standards for Foods for Special Dietary Use for Persons Intolerant to Gluten." Codex Alimentarius. 1979, amended 1983, revised 2008. Accessed August 2013. http://www.codexalimentarius.org/input/download/standards/291/cxs_118e.pdf

11 "Official USDA Food Plans: Cost of Food at Home for Four Levels, U.S. Average, May 2013." U.S. Department of Agriculture, Center for Nutrition Policy and Promotion. June 2013. Accessed August 2013. http://www.cnpp.usda.gov/Publications/FoodPlans/2013/CostofFoodMay2013.pdf

12 "Economic burden of a gluten-free diet." *Journal of Human Nutrition and Dietetics.* October 2007, 20(5): 423–430.
      "Gluten-Free and Regular Foods: A Cost Comparison." *Canadian Journal of Dietetic Practice and Research.* Fall 2008, 69(3): 147–150.
      "Limited availability and higher cost of gluten-free foods." *Journal of Human Nutrition and Dietetics.* October 2011, 24(5): 479–486.

13 "How Much is the Gluten-Free Tax Deduction Really Worth?" *No Gluten, No Problem.* January 29, 2013. Accessed August 2013. http://noglutennoproblem.blogspot.com/2013/01/how-much-is-gluten-free-tax-deduction.html

14 "Store-bought vs. From Scratch: The Cost of Gluten-Free Baked Goods." *No Gluten, No Problem.* February 13, 2013. Accessed August 2013. http://noglutennoproblem.blogspot.com/2013/02/store-bought-vs-from-scratch-cost-of.html

15 "The Gluten-Free Tax Write-Off, and Why It's Flawed." *No Gluten, No Problem.* January 24, 2013. Accessed August 2013. http://noglutennoproblem.blogspot.com/2013/01/the-gluten-free-tax-write-off-and-why.html

16 "Wasted: How America Is Losing Up to 40 Percent of Its Food from Farm to Fork to Landfill." Natural Resources Defense Council. August 2012. Accessed August 2013. http://www.nrdc.org/food/files/wasted-food-IP.pdf

17 "Peak Meat: U.S. Meat Consumption Falling." Earth Policy Institute. March 7, 2012. Accessed August 2013. http://www.earth-policy.org/data_highlights/2012/highlights25

18 "Consumers Speak About Chicken Breast Meat/Breast Tenders Survey Results 2012." National Chicken Council. July 2012. Accessed August 2013. http://www.nationalchickencouncil.org/wp-content/uploads/2012/08/2012-NCC-Consumer-Survey.pdf

19 "Executive Summary: EWG's 2013 Shopper's Guide to Pesticides in Produce." Environmental Working Group. Accessed August 2013. http://www.ewg.org/foodnews/summary.php

20 "Food Choices and Diet Costs: an Economic Analysis." *The Journal of Nutrition.* April 1, 2005. 135(4): 900–904.

21 "Profiling Food Consumption in America." *Agriculture Fact Book.* U.S. Department of Agriculture. Accessed August 2013. http://www.usda.gov/factbook/chapter2.pdf

22 "News Flash: A Healthy Home-Cooked Meal Costs Less Than Fast Food."
    TIME. September 26, 2011. Accessed August 2013. http://business.time
    .com/2011/09/26/news-flash-a-healthy-home-cooked-meal-costs-less-than-
    fast-food/

23 "Boomers Increase Restaurant Visits While Millenials Cut Back, Reports NPD."
    The NPG Group. January 15, 2013. Accessed August 2013. https://www.npd.
    com/wps/portal/npd/us/news/press-releases/boomers-increase-restaurant
    -visits-while-millennials-cut-back-reports-npd/
        "Reservation Nation? Despite Recession, Americans Eat Whopping 250
    Restaurant Meals Per Year, Says LivingSocial Dining Survey." PR Newswire.
    September 15, 2011. Accessed August 2013. https://www.npd.com/wps/portal/
    npd/us/news/press-releases/boomers-increase-restaurant-visits-while-millennials
    -cut-back-reports-npd/

24 "2013 Restaurant Industry Pocket Factbook." National Restaurant Association.
    Accessed August 2013. http://www.restaurant.org/Downloads/PDFs/
    News-Research/Factbook2013_LetterSize.pdf

25 "Consumer Expenditures in 2011." U.S. Bureau of Labor Statistics. April 2013.
    Accessed August 2013. http://www.bls.gov/cex/csxann11.pdf

26 "Gluten-Free Takeout: Which Cities Have the Most G-Free Friendly Restau-
    rants?" *Huffington Post*. July 16, 2013. Accessed August 2013. http://www
    .huffingtonpost.com/2013/07/16/glutenfree-takeout-which-_n_3599652.html

27 "Economic burden of a gluten-free diet." *Journal of Human Nutrition and
    Dietetics*. October 2007, 20(5): 423–430.
        "Limited availability and higher cost of gluten-free foods." *Journal of Hu-
    man Nutrition and Dietetics*. October 2011, 24(5): 479–486.

28 "Do the Poor Pay More for Food? An Analysis of Grocery Store Availability
    and Food Price Disparities." *Journal of Consumer Affairs*. Winter 1999, 33(2):
    276–296.
        "Food store availability and neighborhood characteristics in the United
    States." *Preventive Medicine*. March 2007, 44(3): 189–195.
        "Food Store Types, Availability, and Cost of Foods in a Rural Environ-
    ment." *Journal of the American Dietetic Association*. November 2007, 107(11):
    1916–1923.

29 "The Great Gluten-Free All-Purpose Flour Blend Nutritional Comparison." *No
    Gluten, No Problem*. January 19, 2011. Accessed November 2013. http://noglu-
    tennoproblem.blogspot.com/2011/01/great-gluten-free-all-purpose-flour.html

30 "Ingredient and labeling issues associated with allergenic foods." *Allergy*. April
    2001, 56(s67): 64–69.

31 "Coco-not?" *No Gluten, No Problem*. February 23, 2011. Accessed August 2013.
    http://noglutennoproblem.blogspot.com/2011/02/coco-not.html

ACKNOWLEDGMENTS

FIRST AND FOREMOST, a huge thank you to our daughters, Marin and Charlotte. Whether in our kitchen at home or around the campfire while camping, your eagerness to help with cooking and baking has been a joy. From dicing tofu to measuring flour to being ever-willing taste testers who give brutally honest yet specific, valuable, and insightful feedback, we couldn't have done this book without you. And to Timothy, who was a "(gluten-free) bun in the oven" and then newborn as we finalized this book—we're so happy you too could be part of this book's journey.

To our family and friends, thank you for your continued support, and especially your willingness to taste test iterations of recipes as we honed in on the final version.

To our agent, Jenni Ferrari-Adler, and everyone we've worked with at The Experiment—especially Matthew, Molly, Karen, Cara, Anne, Sarah, and Jack—it's been a pleasure to continue this journey together with you.

And to our readers, many of whom are parents who've contacted us about feeding their gluten-free children, this book is for you. You are the real inspiration and motivation behind it.

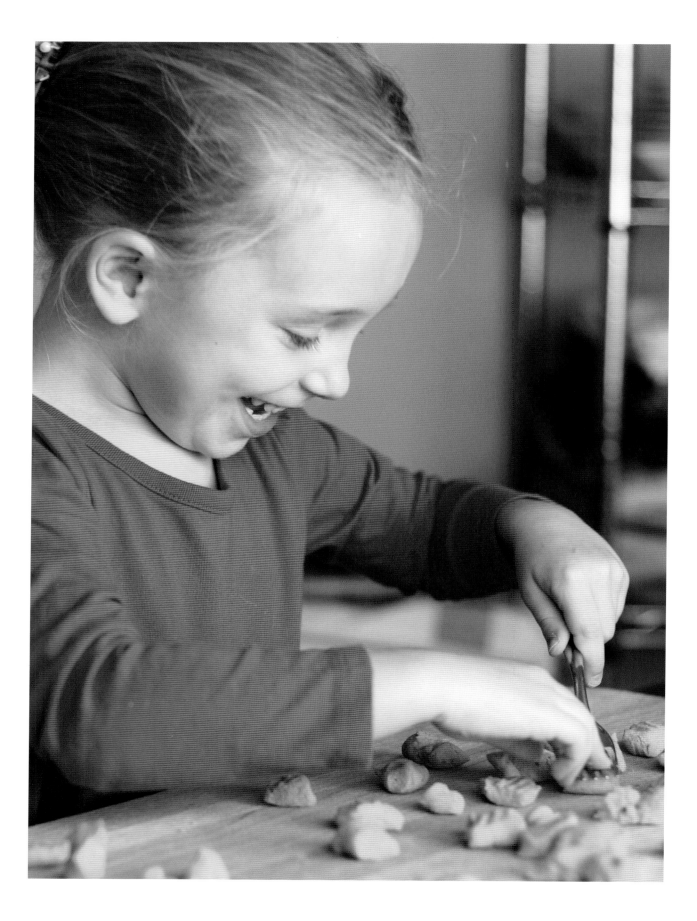

INDEX

ABOUT THE
AUTHORS

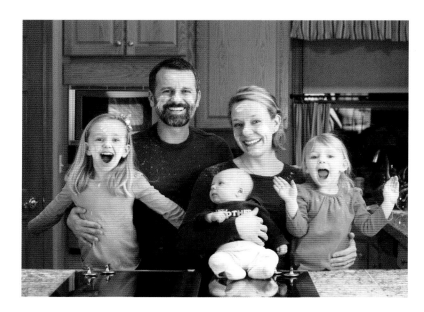

HUSBAND AND WIFE team Kelli and Peter Bronski are also the coauthors of *Artisanal Gluten-Free Cooking* (The Experiment, 2009, 2012) and *Artisanal Gluten-Free Cupcakes* (The Experiment, 2011). *Publishers Weekly* praised *Artisanal Gluten-Free Cooking*'s first edition in a starred review as an "essential horizon-broadening tool for those off gluten." More recently, *Delicious Living* magazine named the revised and updated second edition to its list of "7 great gluten-free cookbooks from 2012," noting that the book "maintains its must-have status."

Kelli and Pete are cofounders of the acclaimed blog *No Gluten, No Problem,* which *The Kitchn* included in its list of "10 Inspiring Blogs for Gluten-Free Food & Cooking," noting the couple's "thorough and lucid writing." Triumph Dining also nominated *No Gluten, No Problem* for 'best gluten-free blog" in its 2013 The Best of Gluten-Free Awards and Healthline.com named it one of the "best allergy blogs of 2013." The blog focuses on diverse from-scratch recipes, in-depth gluten-free reporting, and tips for living a happy, healthy, and active gluten-free lifestyle. Their recipes have been cited in venues ranging from the *Washington Post* to *The Food Network* blog.

Kelli is a food and hospitality industry veteran, having graduated from Cornell University's prestigious School of Hotel Administration. She spent nearly a decade with Hilton, including at the Waldorf=Astoria Hotel in New York City, and earned the company's Circle of Excellence honor. Her lifelong passion for cooking and baking dates back to the early days of her childhood spent in the kitchen with her grandmother.

Pete is an award-winning writer whose work has appeared in more than eighty magazines, including *National Geographic Traveler, Men's Journal, Relish,* and *Edible Front Range,* and is the editorial director of a nonprofit think tank. He is also the author of four other books in addition to the couple's cookbooks, including *The Gluten-Free Edge: A Nutrition and Training Guide for Peak Athletic Performance and an Active Gluten-Free Life* (The Experiment, 2012, coauthored with Melissa McLean Jory, MNT). A spokesperson for the National Foundation for Celiac Awareness as one of the organization's Athletes for Awareness, Pete is an endurance athlete focused on mountain/trail ultramarathons.

Kelli and Pete have been gluten-free since January 2007, when Pete was de facto diagnosed with celiac disease. They maintain a 100 percent gluten-free home, where every recipe must please the palates of their children, Marin, Charlotte, and Timothy.

Together, Kelli and Pete have taught gluten-free cooking demos, seminars, and webinars for organizations including the Gluten & Allergen Free Expo, Gluten-Free Culinary Summit, Whole Foods, ShopRite, and regional celiac and gluten intolerance support groups. They have been featured in publications such as *Allergic Living, Gluten-Free Living,* the *Daily Camera* (Boulder, CO), *Poughkeepsie Journal* (NY), and *Edible Front Range;* appeared on Denver's NBC television affiliate; and been interviewed on National Public Radio's *The Splendid Table.*

Both New York natives, they now live in Colorado.

For more information, visit them online: nogluten-noproblem.com

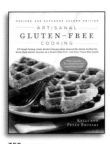

352 pages
Color photos throughout
$21.95
Paperback:
   978-1-61519-050-8
Ebook: 978-1-61519-157-4

Artisanal Gluten-Free Cooking

275 Great-Tasting, From-Scratch Recipes from Around the World, Perfect for Every Meal and for Anyone on a Gluten-Free Diet—and Even Those Who Aren't

Since *Artisanal Gluten-Free Cooking*'s original publication in 2009, more and more home cooks have embraced Kelli and Peter Bronski's high-quality, from-scratch gluten-free recipes for every meal. This revised and expanded second edition is better than ever, with a thorough introduction to gluten-free shopping and cooking, an expanded array of vegetarian options, and dozens of globally inspired recipes, from bagels to birthday cake, perfectly suited to the Bronskis' signature all-purpose flour blend—including Belgian Waffles, Garlic Naan, pizzas and pastas galore, Cannoli, Carrot Cake, Blueberry Pie, cookies, and much more.

"An essential, horizon-broadening tool for those off gluten."
—*Publishers Weekly* (starred review)

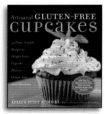

272 pages
Color photos throughout
$16.95
Paperback:
   978-1-61519-036-2
Ebook: 978-1-61519-136-9

Artisanal Gluten-Free Cupcakes

50 From-Scratch Recipes to Delight Every Cupcake Devotee—Gluten-Free and Otherwise

The wait for an entire cookbook of gluten-free cupcakes is over! In *Artisanal Gluten-Free Cupcakes*, the Bronskis bring their accessible but "artisanal" approach to these inventive homemade cupcakes. The bakery-quality confections include kid-pleasing favorites like Vanilla Cupcakes with Chocolate Frosting or "Peanut Butter Cup" Cakes, as well as subtle and surprising treats like Mojito or Poached Pearfection cupcakes. With tips for making egg-, dairy-, and refined-sugar-free versions, these are cupcakes so good even those who eat gluten will love them.

"Our gluten-free world just got a whole lot sweeter
with Kelli and Peter's amazing new book on cupcakes."
—Carol Fenster, award-winning author of
100 Best Gluten-Free Recipes

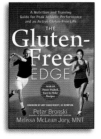

384 pages
$15.95
Paperback:
   978-1-61519-052-2
Ebook: 978-1-61519-149-9

The Gluten-Free Edge

A Nutrition and Training Guide for Peak Athletic Performance and an Active Gluten-Free Life
by Peter Bronski and Melissa McLean Jory, MNT

The Gluten-Free Edge is the first comprehensive resource for athletes with celiac disease or gluten sensitivity. The book covers:

- What to eat during training, competition, and recovery
- How to deal with group meals, eating on the road, and getting "glutened"
- Insights from prominent athletes already living the gluten-free edge
- And 50 simple, high-octane recipes to fuel your performance.

"A great book for both the weekend warrior and the professional."
—Bruce Gordon, marathon swimmer and
the first person to swim the 18 miles across Lake Coeur d'Alene